Living with Hypopituitarism

and other things that happened to come along

MARILYN HARVEY

i

First published in Great Britain in 2017

CreateSpace

British Library Cataloguing-in-Publication Data

A catalogue record for this book is available from the British Library

ISBN-13 978-1973933700

ISBN-10 1973933705

Thank you to my wonderful family and friends for all your love and support

Acknowledgements

The Pituitary Foundation

Dr J K Powrie MD FRCP

Doctors, surgeons and therapists who have treated me over the years.

Dr Andrea Kay BA PhD, for editing my book

All proceeds from the sale of this book go to The Pituitary Foundation. Thank you.

Correspondence

marilyn.harvey3@gmail.com

Contents

Note to the reader

This is not a medical book and is not intended to replace advice from your doctor. Do not make changes to your prescribed medications without advice from your doctor and do not try taking any medicine that hasn't been prescribed by your doctor.

Introduction

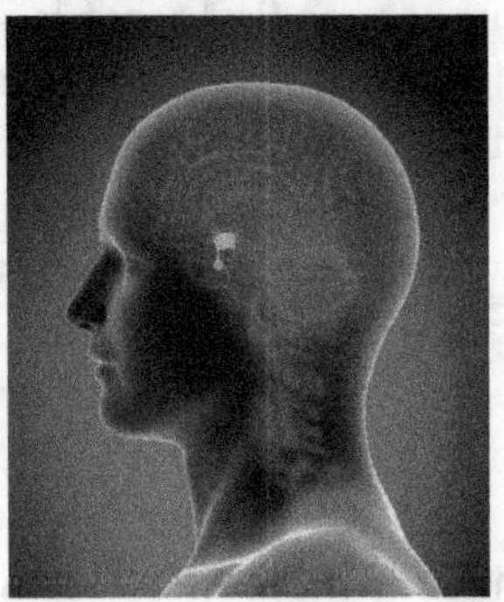

Image courtesy of The Pituitary Foundation

It must have been at least fifteen years ago when an acupuncturist I was visiting for treatment for back pain suggested I write a book about my unusual medical history. At the time I didn't think anyone would be that interested in my story; neither was I sure I wanted to commit myself to such an undertaking.

Fast forward to last year, 2016. During my six-monthly check-up with my endocrinologist, I was given the startling news that the result of a recent bone density scan showed my T-scores were −2.5 in my lumbar spine and −2.9 in my left forearm, indicating that these were now in the osteoporotic range. We had hoped for a better result, especially as I had been taking growth hormone for four years.

As I sat waiting for a routine blood test following my consultation, it was difficult to clear my head. How had I got here? What had caused this to happen? Many questions needed answers, each one taking me back to the possible, or even very plausible trigger for the eventual weakening of my bones: a pituitary apoplexy in 1972 which, almost as long as ten years later, had finally led to a diagnosis of hypopituitarism. It occurred to me as I sat there that this was probably the right time to start writing that book!

I have combed through medical records as well as my diaries, carried out a little research and asked questions of my endocrinologist. But, this isn't just an account of doctors' letters, diagnoses and treatments about my condition and other things that happened to come along. It is about my personal journey; one that has certainly been interesting and not lacking in surprises! Many years of physical, mental and emotional challenges have brought with them a search for, if not possible solutions, ways, at least, of dealing with the difficulties they present, all of which have enabled me to come to terms with and learn from my experiences.

So here it is, for those who have hypopituitarism or any other pituitary condition, or indeed anyone interested in my story. I have read many accounts written by pituitary patients in The Pituitary Foundation's magazine, *Pituitary Life*. These people courageously describe the many life changes and challenges a pituitary condition presents. I hope you find this story of my journey as encouraging as I have found theirs.

1

In the beginning

The good physician treats the disease; the great physician treats the patient who has the disease
William Osler

This was no hangover. Attempts to open my eyes were thwarted by the excruciating pain in my head, which seemed to fill my entire being. Each time I recall that day, I'm taken back to a darkened room, shadows of various sizes of furniture silhouetted against the walls and my drunken efforts to get out of bed and reach the telephone. I needed to let my office know I thought I had a migraine so wouldn't be turning up. Having experienced migraines before, I believed I was having yet another and assumed it would pass in a day or so. Somehow I managed to make the call, swallowed some pain killers and fell, like a brick, back into bed.

It was a Thursday in November, 1972. I was twenty-four years old and living in an airy bedsit in a large Georgian-style house in south-east London, overlooking beautiful green spaces. After enjoying the absolute freedom of living and travelling for two and a half years in Canada and the USA, then backpacking around Europe for a short time, I had finally decided to settle in London once more where I would be near family and friends. Work in the City was abundant in those days so I was able to find secretarial posts with ease by working for various agencies, picking and choosing depending on the hourly rate and nature of the job.

The day wore on. As I drifted in and out of consciousness, the weak November light that had seeped through gaps in the heavy curtains gradually began to fade. Night was approaching when the telephone rang and I thought it would stop before I could get to it, but thankfully the ringing persisted. On the other end of the line I heard the muffled sound of my boyfriend's voice and after listening to my attempts at explaining my predicament, he said he would be round. It didn't seem too long before his large frame appeared in the doorway of my room and, after taking one look at my prostrate form on the bed, he called a doctor.

I can't quite remember what was prescribed or advised but, whatever it was, it had no effect. It must have been the following evening when another doctor was called. She quickly scribbled a prescription for sleeping tablets. It struck me much later that this seemed an odd thing to give someone suffering from a blinding headache, increasing neck pain and intolerance to light. Maybe it was because I happened to mention that I had trouble sleeping because of the pain! I never discovered why my own GP failed to turn up but maybe it was because the calls for help were made at unsociable hours. In the meantime the pain grew and grew in intensity and, as it grew, the dull, sickening sensation developed in my neck making it difficult for me to move my head.

The sleeping pills took me into the darkness of oblivion but, on waking, I discovered that the pain remained. My head continued to throb, rather like the pulsating sound of an engine, reminding me of those I used to be a little afraid of as a child, growing up in the north-east of England. The engines that beat and churned in the depths below the water company pumping station, outside which my brother and I played, only a stone's throw away from our aunt's house where we had been born. Later, I would sometimes dream of those cylindrical metal dinosaurs churning, sucking me downwards into the whirling green waters beneath the ground.

I was under the impression that it was the following morning when I became vaguely aware of the telephone ringing again. It rang relentlessly so I struggled, through the painful darkness in my head, towards the receiver. There followed a strange and disjointed conversation with said boyfriend revealing that, rather than spending the previous night in deep slumber, I had actually slept through two nights. The realisation that an entire day had been erased from my life left me feeling vaguely perplexed yet quite unable to react.

By now the pain in my neck was worsening considerably, possibly because I had made the effort to get out of bed to answer the telephone. Once back in bed it became almost impossible for me to lift myself up and as the pain gradually dulled my senses it became me and I became the pain. We were one mass; a deepening, throbbing, sickening darkness was taking over, assuming control.

It seemed quite out of character for a seemingly detached boyfriend to suddenly appear almost as soon as I had put down the receiver. It was now Sunday and another doctor was called. This time a man of action breezed in and, after asking me to raise each leg and sit up, both of which were impossible, then examining my eyes, he told me he suspected that I might have meningitis. I feebly asked this wonderfully efficient medicine man to explain what this meant and he did so, although I don't know whether or not I took in the implications of his diagnosis. I listened as he picked up the telephone and called an ambulance, asking for me to be transported to St Bartholomew's hospital in London. In no time at all, two paramedics were manoeuvring me into a wheelchair, then into the waiting ambulance. The sirens yelled and, at every turn the ambulance made, my head and neck screamed in protest.

On a trolley, up in a lift and into a room which, I later learned, was just off a main ward. My boyfriend had left by now but I have a vague recollection of two people standing at the end of my bed looking down at me. One a woman, dazed and distraught, the other a man, detached yet pale. My parents. My mother remembers a small, darkened room illuminated with only the faintest blue light and it was in this room that I was to have a lumbar puncture.

There must be a number of nurses out there with very sore hands or crushed finger bones after patients such as myself have held on to them to help endure the sickening sensation and pain of needles sinking into one's lumbar region! I gratefully squeezed the hand of a young nurse when she offered it to me and at the same time sunk my teeth into the pillow.

Soon afterwards the doctors came to tell me that the result of the lumbar puncture showed I probably had meningism. The easiest way to describe this condition is to say that symptoms of meningism mimic those of meningitis; for example, neck stiffness, headache, intolerance to bright lights, but it is caused by irritation rather than inflammation of the meninges, or protective membranes covering the brain and spinal cord. It was to be some years before this diagnosis was revised.

Medication followed diagnosis before I was moved out of the airless side room and into a huge ward belonging to the Victorian era where rows of occupied beds seemed to stretch forever. Such vast, impersonal wards are now, thankfully, a thing of the past. Nurses seemed to buzz around in all directions yet still managed to give excellent care. However, just before I was moved from my room I experienced a somewhat frosty natured ward sister who told me to sit upright with the support of two pillows. Despite my protestations that it hurt my neck to sit up she insisted, saying that the consultant was about to do his rounds! As soon as she left the room I resumed my supine position. The consultant didn't seem at all bothered.

'It's lifting,' I heard the doctor say, but the horror of the hallucinations, brought on no doubt by the medication I had been given, wasn't lifting. The human skulls continued to glare, hollow-eyed at me. What could they see, lying there in their ghastly pit, glaring from their deep, dark empty sockets? Pile upon pile of wasted, colourless bones lay scattered on stone ground. Hollow, sunken eye spaces stared upwards as I flew above them on my vividly coloured, patterned carpet. Swooping then diving, only just missing those dry and lifeless bones before taking off and rising into an orange foam sky. As I opened my eyes the nightmare vanished but was back again as soon as they closed, then gone again as they opened once more until I wondered which state was the true reality. It must have been the one where I heard a voice calling my name, the one where I could view the normality of the hospital ward from behind my dark glasses. Silly, children's plastic red-framed sunglasses, found at the last minute, protecting my eyes from the light.

The exhausted doctor on his daily rounds, stethoscope askew, seemed unperturbed when I related my experiences, while the eyebrows of the young nurse accompanying him almost rose to meet her hairline. Over the course of a few days, the 'trips' gradually faded and disappeared. I cheered up as visitors came and went but left hospital after a few days feeling I had visited a strange place, a place that had taken part of me away and which would take some time to restore. It took at least two months before I felt well enough to go back to the office where I worked or to enjoy a normal diet. Much to the amusement of my boyfriend, I had cravings for milk and a well-known stout which lasted for a few weeks. The doctor at St Bartholomew's, who I saw on my review day, didn't seem to be concerned at all by this and discharged me.

During the years that followed and despite noticing a developing tiredness and difficulty socialising, I put one career behind me and embraced another by leaving the world of commerce and entering the teaching profession. I was drawn to teaching after being introduced to a class at the special needs school where a friend taught. Her enthusiasm for her work was contagious. Besides, I was becoming rather disillusioned with my work as a secretary in the City and wanted to do something more meaningful with my life. So, I started studying at a teacher training college in Deptford, London, which soon became part of Goldsmiths College before being demolished many years later and replaced by blocks of flats. While studying there from 1976 to 1979, I was beginning to notice a further decline in my energy and found I was battling with the ability to concentrate and complete tasks. Socialising with friends was an effort. I even resorted to drinking small quantities of fortified red wine to try to boost my iron levels, but to no avail – although the effects were quite pleasant! My moods would change uncharacteristically as the tiredness encroached more and more on my life. Despite my efforts to discover why, I would have to wait some years before the medical profession could provide me with an explanation for the changes that were taking place.

By September 1979 I was teaching in an inner London primary school so put the increasing tiredness down to the nature of the job. Who wouldn't? Teaching and tiredness are synonymous, are they not? Then there was the coldness and the shivering. I'd wonder why I needed to add extra layers of clothing when the temperature was not especially low or why I looked so pale. Yet during holiday periods I was under the illusion that I must be in good health and just needed a break and some sunshine. So, that year I travelled to Canada and America enjoying visiting old friends and in 1980 I took a holiday in sunny Greece. The breaks were relaxing and distracted me somewhat from my difficulties. I wonder if I was probably in denial. I was getting on with my life when perhaps I should have been listening to the warning signs and taking more determined steps to find out what was going on.

Then, one day in the autumn of 1980, my mother was visiting as I was quite ill and unable to move much at all. She called my GP and he arranged for an ambulance to take me back to St Bartholomew's. Blood tests were taken but I was simply told that

I didn't have what I'd had in 1972 and could go home! As we waited for a taxi my mother and I looked at each other in disbelief. I wondered whether I was wasting everyone's time.

On reflection, I can see that changes in my appearance were developing insidiously. I lost a lot of weight and friends began to comment on how pale I looked. I was beginning to notice an even greater lethargy and a struggle to complete tasks such as the work required to complete a Bachelor of Education degree. This was a time when the Department of Education encouraged teachers to reach degree level. So, to safeguard future employment, I felt somewhat pressured to improve my qualifications. I was studying part time and attending evening classes which meant my work at a local primary school began to suffer. It bothered me that displays were rushed and my lesson preparation seemed less efficient. In the meantime, and despite everything that was going on, I met Louis and we married in February 1981. Even today, my close friends remark on how pale I looked on my wedding day.

Another missed opportunity to discover why I was experiencing such unusual tiredness, feeling cold and generally battling to get through the day, occurred in June 1981 when a technician at the pathology laboratory at my local hospital spotted something! My GP had ordered a blood test, the result of which suggested I may have the condition 'hypopituitarism'. I remember him shaking his head as he read this report to me but, nevertheless, he referred me to King's College Hospital. All I can find in my medical records, dated August 1981, is a note that an endocrinologist at King's felt I was lacking hydrocortisone but I don't remember, and can't find, reference to any further investigations.

In a remarkably short space of time further physical changes began to make themselves obvious. As the tiredness increased, my hair became drier and photographs taken on holiday in the summer of 1981 show that I was developing a fuller face. Not only was my face becoming rounder but it was developing a faint yellow hue which lasted for a while. It is a mystery why this occurred but I was later to learn from my endocrinologist that the facial swelling was due to fluid retention because of low levels of the thyroid hormone. The photographs below show the changes that took place between February 1981 and July 1982.

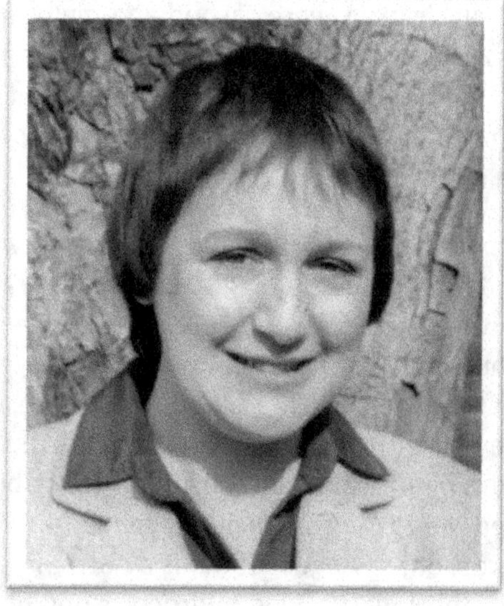

14 February 1981. My wedding day when signs of a fuller face were just beginning to show

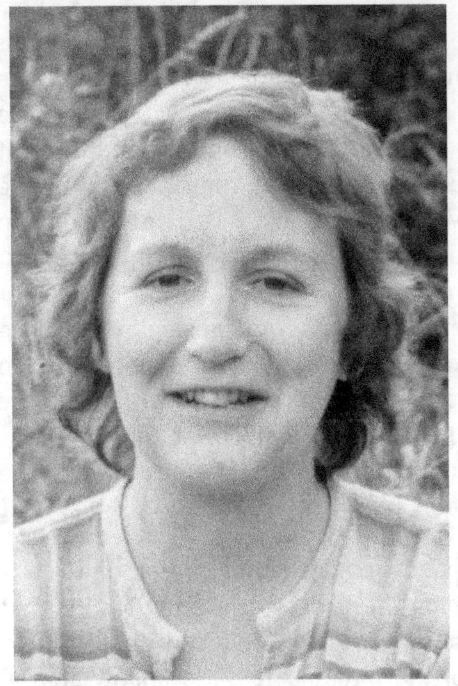

August 1981, when I was developing a rounder face

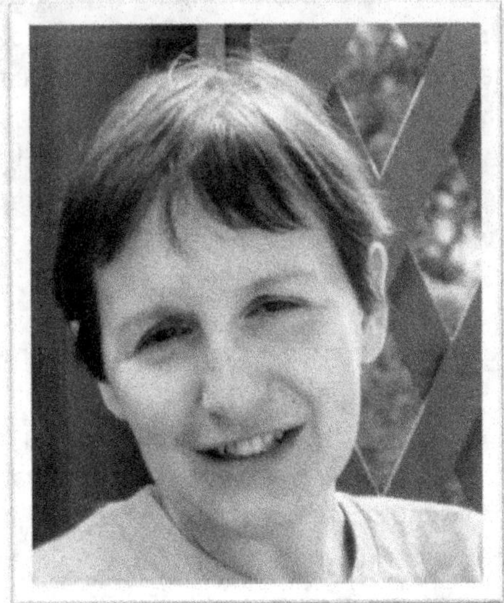

July 1982. After three months of hormone replacement, I am looking much healthier and my face has regained its shape

Shortly after the second photograph was taken I took a serious look at myself in the mirror and thought it was time to take decisive action. I had not had a period for two years since stopping the contraceptive pill for the second time and thought it reasonable to use the desire to become pregnant as an excuse to get to the bottom of what was going on. Perhaps I had been under the impression that it took the body some time to adjust to a normal menstrual cycle after a woman has taken the pill for some years, but waiting for two years for changes to take place began to seem rather extreme. Louis and I were quite sure we would love to have children at some point but it seemed that the only way forward was to give the impression that our desire was an immediate one. I talked to my GP and was referred to the Gynaecology House Surgeon at King's.

My medical records show I reported that I'd had one year's amenorrhoea after stopping the contraceptive pill for the first time in 1978. At King's, in February 1979, investigations showed that although an X-ray of the pituitary fossa (a hollow area in which the pituitary gland sits) was normal my serum progesterone was low. I decided at the time to leave further tests and treatment in abeyance and was invited to contact the team when I wanted to take investigations further. Maybe I should have pursued matters then instead of resuming taking the pill as it was obvious something wasn't as it should be. At least I was getting some oestrogen which would have been protecting my bones

Most, but sadly not all, doctors have a tactful manner or appropriate compassion. 'Some women would be glad not to have periods' is a remark made by the examining doctor on my visit to King's in October 1981, which will stay with me always. Some women? Show me a woman of thirty-three who would not be concerned that she was suffering from amenorrhoea. I made further visits to King's College Hospital before I was prescribed 75 mg of Clomid which, I was told by a very confident doctor, would restore my periods by stimulating ovulation. Upon being informed a few weeks later that it had not done its magic, a rather surprised and slightly flustered doctor referred me to the Gynaecology House Surgeon who wrote to my GP to say I was being referred to the Infertility Clinic. This was followed by a further letter from the Gynaecological Registrar in January 1982 stating that I would be having further hormone investigations then, in a letter to my GP the following month, he wrote:

> The latest results on Mrs Harvey are suggestive of
> secondary hypothyroidism with primary infertility. I
> am referring her to the endocrine clinic.

Then things really started moving. After examining me and asking various questions, the endocrinologist, who I will refer to as Dr L, suspected that something serious was going on. He described the condition as 'life threatening but treatable', although at the time didn't give it a name. Within a few days I was despatched to BUPA for a CT scan. Louis came with me and waited while I was directed to a room where I had my scan. I remember lying down with my head in a tunnel aware of lights flashing around me as a whirring sound pervaded my ear drums. I was given an intravenous injection of a contrast dye, used to highlight specific areas of the brain. This made me feel quite sick and my head objected to the pain it caused.

Within a few days I was back at King's, face to face with Dr L, the endocrinologist and was admitted to hospital for further tests, mainly to see how much hydrocortisone I needed. During this time the days dragged on and not much happened apart from the odd blood test. I was even sent home for a weekend. While I was in hospital, one very kind doctor listened to my concern about continuing with my B.Ed. degree and wrote a letter to give to the examiners stating that, because of my condition, my concentration would be impaired. I was very grateful for this support. In contrast, a comment made by a junior doctor, who declared that I wouldn't be able to have children, really surprised me! Fortunately, I was able to counter his remark immediately as Dr L had told me earlier that, with fertility treatment, I should be able to conceive one day.

My GP received a letter from Dr L in early March in which he describes me as almost certainly panhypopituitary. It appeared that the cranial scan I'd had at BUPA revealed atrophy of the anterior lobe of my pituitary gland, possibly caused by an apoplexy in 1972 and resulting in hypopituitarism. He prescribed hydrocortisone tablets, 20 mg in the morning and 10 mg in the evening for the time being. Here is an extract from a report written around the same time by the Senior Medical Registrar:

> Investigations as an outpatient had suggested pituitary insufficiency. On examination she was pale with a face consistent with hypopituitarism … Investigations: CT scan of the pituitary fossa showed that the basal cisterns extend into the upper two-thirds of the pituitary fossa outlining the pituitary stalk. The appearances were of a partially empty sella. This lady demonstrates some features of hypopituitarism particularly the low T4 [the T4 test is used to evaluate thyroid function] and the amenorrhoea with low gonadotrophin levels [hormones secreted by the pituitary to stimulate the ovaries]. It is possible this is consequent upon an episode of pituitary apoplexy when she had the headaches in 1972. In order for her to become pregnant she will require HMG/HCG [fertility] treatment. It may be advisable to treat her with oestrogens alone for a short period before attempting to induce ovulation. She is therefore being seen in the Gynaecology Clinic and in the Endocrinology Clinic.

Now I had a clearer picture of what had caused the anterior lobe of my pituitary gland to atrophy. According to Wikipedia:

> The causes of a pituitary apoplexy can be bleeding into the pituitary or, [as in my case], by blocked blood flow

of the pituitary.

This is what the doctor believed had happened. Certainly, the symptoms I experienced in 1972 matched those associated with a pituitary apoplexy; for example, headache, light sensitivity, nausea, and neck rigidity.

You may recall that it was thought I had suffered from meningism in 1972 and I wondered whether my new diagnosis of a pituitary apoplexy in any way resembled symptoms of the previous diagnosis. I was very interested to discover that:

> The diagnosis of pituitary apoplexy is often delayed as
> ~80% of these patients will have no previous history of
> a pituitary problem and the clinical features mimic
> other more common neurological conditions.[1]

This source also reports that a diagnosis of a pituitary problem should be considered in patients who have, among other symptoms, acute severe headache, photophobia, neck stiffness and signs of meningitis!

In April 1982 I was seen by the Lecturer in Obstetrics and Gynaecology at King's, who I will refer to as Mr W. I find the following extract from a copy of his letter to the Senior Medical Registrar, most relevant.

> I have had a long discussion with this patient
> concerning the long-term adverse effects of
> oestrogen-deficiency in terms of changes in lipid and
> bone status.

He prescribed oestrone sulphate (Harmogen) 3 mg daily continuously and Provera (progesterone) 2.5 mg daily for the first twelve days of each calendar month.

Mr W wrote to the Senior Medical Registrar informing him of his findings and I vaguely remember having a consultation with this man when I was told I had adequate ACTH reserves (ACTH, normally produced by the pituitary gland, stimulates the production and release of cortisol from the adrenal gland) and could stop taking my hydrocortisone tablets. He increased my thyroxine to 150 micrograms daily. My medical records confirm this in a letter dated 21 April 1982.

My next review with Mr W was in July when he advised me to continue with my present medication of oestrone sulphate and Provera. Also that month I saw Dr L and reported feeling unwell, experiencing frequent sore throats, general tiredness and malaise. He informed my GP that:

> I would have expected this lady to be adrenal
> insufficient as she was both hypothyroid and
> gonadotrophin deficient. Although our biochemical
> tests showed that she was able to produce adequate
> levels of cortisol I am still a bit suspicious and have,
> therefore, asked her to increase the dose of
> hydrocortisone to 10 mg in the morning and 5 mg in
> the afternoon.

September arrived and another consultation with Dr L. This time I was happy to report I felt quite well although I was experiencing some swelling of the lymph nodes. Dr L decided I needed more hydrocortisone and increased my dose to 20 mg in the morning and 10 mg in the afternoon. I have remained on a daily dose of 30 mg hydrocortisone ever since.

A further appointment with Mr W in the same month confirmed that I was extremely well and had no symptoms of oestrogen deficiency. Following my request, he put my name on the waiting list to attend the infertility clinic for HMG (human menopausal gonadotropin) and HCG (human chorionic gonadotropin) cyclical therapy.

So what is hypopituitarism? I had no idea at the time but later found the following useful description:

> The pituitary gland produces a number of hormones
> or chemicals which are released into the blood to
> control other glands in the body. If the pituitary is not
> producing one or more of these hormones or not
> producing enough then this condition is known as
> hypopituitarism.[2]

Maybe it would be helpful to take a brief look at the hormone replacement I was prescribed.

It was explained to me after diagnosis that hydrocortisone is a steroid hormone, produced by the adrenal glands, which are situated at the top of each kidney and is essential for survival. The inner section of each adrenal gland (medulla) produces adrenalin which is part of the fight or flight response when we are under stress; for example, when you mistake a coil of rope in the path in front of you for a snake or, much worse, are involved in an accident. The outer section (cortex) releases hormones, one of which is cortisol (known as hydrocortisone when used as a medication); cortisol helps the body deal with stress, controls blood pressure and circulation and blood sugar levels. Wikipedia explains that the adrenal glands are typically the first to be affected in a pituitary apoplexy and cease to produce cortisol although my current endocrinologist explained that, depending on the intensity of the apoplexy, all hormones are likely to be affected.

Despite the Senior Medical Registrar's earlier findings, I was prescribed hydrocortisone replacement therapy. This corticosteroid (steroid) replacement is also taken in cases of Addison's disease when the adrenal gland fails to produce cortisol.

Thyroxine is produced by the thyroid gland, which sits on the front of the neck under the skin and muscle. Thyroxine plays a crucial role in metabolism, heart and digestive function, brain development, bone health and muscle control. It was interesting to learn from my endocrinologist that too much thyroxine, rather than too little, causes osteoporosis.

Oestrogen is of course the female hormone. It is released by the ovaries and helps to release eggs from the ovaries as well as regulating a woman's periods. One of its main functions is to control bone density. It is well reported that problems caused by a reduction in oestrogen include bone thinning which can lead to osteoporosis and fractures. The main role of progesterone, which is also released by the ovaries, is to prepare the lining of the uterus for pregnancy. In men, testosterone replacement is used.

In the days that followed my diagnosis, I tried not to dwell on the many questions filling my head such as why the medical profession hadn't suspected a pituitary condition earlier, although I do understand that even some of the more experienced doctors may misdiagnose some of the time, especially when working under pressure to see an allotted number of patients in a short period of time. I would not like to think that some of it is due to complacency. The most significant factor, and one that induced some fear, was that my body had been deprived of these essential hormones for almost ten years. What irreparable damage had been done during that time?

As soon as I started taking hormone replacement medication my body reacted differently, particularly to the daily dosage of hydrocortisone. I can only describe this as being on a 'high' for a few days as I could not keep still and my body seemed quite out of control as I rushed everywhere, surprising everyone. I remember putting up a display in my classroom, previously an activity that would have taken much physical effort, but on this occasion I found I had completed the task, quite creatively, in half the time. I can only imagine that this reaction was due to the shock my body must have been experiencing with the reintroduction of a hormone it had been deprived of for so long, or was I over-prescribed?

While coming to terms with having this rare condition, I remembered my GCE Human Anatomy lessons at school when the teacher made reference to the pituitary gland but I didn't really learn much about its essential role at all. What really sticks in my mind from those lessons is the wonderful word 'corticosteroids' with its musical, syllabic sounds. Obviously, I was totally unaware then of just how familiar that word would become in the future! Over the years I have met only a few people who fully understand the role of this tiny gland, or have even heard of its name, unless they are trained medics, know someone who has a pituitary condition or have one themselves. To find out a little more about this amazing gland, please go to the Appendix.

2

Thank you, Pergonal!

The year 1982 ended on an optimistic note. Taking replacement therapy meant that I had more energy and felt in better health. I was excited about the prospect of becoming pregnant as I had commenced treatment at the infertility clinic at King's under the care of Dr S. I'm not sure if the procedure is the same today as it was in the 1980s but it was rather complex then. I was given injections of Pergonal, a combination of human FSH (the follicle-stimulating hormone) and LH (the luteinising hormone). I needed to collect urine then send samples off to a laboratory for testing for the effects of Pergonal. The accuracy of the reading was vital in determining when my injection of HCG was to be given. This injection was given to stimulate the ovary to release an egg as soon as the ovary had produced the appropriate level of oestrogen. On 31 December 1982 I have recorded in my diary that I was given my 'booster' injection – the HCG. I was full of optimism. On 7 January 1983 I saw Dr S again and he was sure that I had ovulated. So we had to wait and see. Everyone at school was interested, especially the headteacher who even joked about me having a water birth in the nursery paddling pool!

For almost two weeks I noticed some subtle changes taking place in my body but then, on 20 January, I discovered I wasn't pregnant and, although this was only our first attempt at using Pergonal, I felt terribly disappointed. Dr S was surprised and even took a blood sample to test for pregnancy anyway but it proved to be negative. Within a few days I came to terms with events and looked ahead to the next cycle.

My diary shows that on 28 January I attended the infertility clinic again and was given my first injection of Pergonal for this new cycle. I had my second Pergonal injection on the 31 January and a scan was taken although there wasn't much to see that day. On the 7 February Dr S decided that I was ready for my 'booster' injection. Here we go again, I thought, but with rather less euphoria this time! I was having to monitor my temperature but after a couple of days I didn't think that I had ovulated as it was still low. Then a few days later, just before my thirty-fifth birthday on 15 February, I found that my temperature had risen so guessed I must have ovulated. On 23 February it had dropped one point and but on 28 February Dr S told me he thought there was a possibility I may be pregnant but we would need to wait another week to be certain. The test I was given was not exactly negative, nor was it positive! It was wait and see time again!

I turned up at King's on 7 March 1983 and after looking at the scan, Dr S gave me the wonderful news that I was pregnant. I remember feeling completely overwhelmed, then, barely feeling my feet on the ground, hurried downstairs to make an appointment with the antenatal clinic. I couldn't wait to phone Louis who was speechless when he heard the news. I wish I could have seen his face! My family and friends were very excited and when I arrived back at school everyone leapt in the air when I gave them the news. They even managed to find a bottle of wine to celebrate! The following day I still couldn't believe that I had this tiny, growing human life inside me. It happens every day, yet to me it was a miracle. My last appointment for a scan was on the 21 March when Dr S gave me a photograph of my tiny embryo, which showed this 'microdot' in its amniotic sac inside my womb. 'Everything is progressing nicely and you should see the end product in early November,' he confirmed. While attending the infertility clinic some of the women I sat waiting with were desperate to have a child and had already attended many sessions at the clinic but without success. The news I was given on this particular day made me aware that, despite my pituitary condition, I was so very fortunate that something could be done and to this day remain extremely grateful for the help and support of Dr S and his team.

In March I visited the antenatal clinic for the first time and everyone was very pleasant and helpful, especially the doctor who took careful note of my pituitary condition and daily medication. However, he seemed doubtful that I would be able to breastfeed as I probably wouldn't produce enough prolactin after delivery. While there I had a scan and saw the amazing sight of my baby's heartbeat. At a later appointment in June, I was seen by Mr W who announced that everything was going well.

As with all pregnancies, I was feeling very tired at times but I had also developed a terrific thirst and was drinking what seemed to be gallons of water each day. Dr L decided I should spend 24 hours in hospital having a water deprivation test as he wanted to check why I needed to drink so much and wondered whether my pituitary may have something to do with it. I was admitted on 28 July and for this test I had to drink lots of water up until 8.30am, then nil by mouth until 4.30pm. During the test I lost some weight but not enough for them to be concerned so it was a relief to know that the posterior part of my pituitary gland wasn't affected. I didn't have diabetes insipidus; I was just thirsty! Unfortunately, most of the time I craved fizzy drinks which I now know were not the healthiest option! I saw Dr L again in September when he reported that he was happy with my progress. I'd had the odd episode of swollen glands when he had advised me to increase my hydrocortisone but, apart from that, he thought I was managing well. I learned then that I would need a 100 mg injection of cortisol when I went into labour to deal with the stress my body would go through during delivery.

Despite an incredibly hot summer that year, which made life very uncomfortable at times, I had a fairly uneventful pregnancy. Baby was moving quite a lot. Not only was this an exciting experience for us but we found it very funny seeing our cat's perplexed expression as she sat on my bump (an evening ritual) probably wondering why she was being gently pummelled from below. Yet, despite this, she never attempted to jump off!

We awaited the delivery date of early November, but baby had other ideas! At around 2am on Wednesday 28 September my waters broke. I wondered whether eating my friend Georgia's bread and butter pudding the previous evening had anything to do with it! I was convinced that I had simply experienced Braxton Hicks contractions (intermittent weak contractions of the uterus) the day before but a friend who was visiting at the time was very doubtful. She was right! A shocked Louis responded in a daze to my cries of 'My waters have broken!' Half asleep, he somehow managed to find the telephone to call the maternity ward at King's. I remember faintly hearing the ward sister's words drifting down the telephone line, 'We'll be seeing you!' By the time we threw things into a bag and drove off, I felt minor contractions starting – this was it, baby was going to surprise us all by arriving five weeks early.

On arrival we found our way through an eerie, dimly lit hospital to maternity admissions. I was examined and monitored for baby's heartbeat then taken to the first stage room by a super midwife where I was given 100 mg of cortisol. The contractions became stronger very quickly so I rested my head against Louis' chest and concentrated on the breathing techniques I had learned at the few National Childbirth Trust classes I had attended. Despite those lessons, Louis had to remind me to flop, relax and breathe as I tensed with pain. My diary notes confirm that I was soon cautiously winding my way down the brightly lit corridor to the delivery room, aware of the yelling and groaning of women in childbirth, followed by the tiny cries of their new born babies as they entered the world. I allowed the doctor and a different midwife, to place a probe over baby's head so they could monitor its progress. As the contractions became incredibly strong, I wondered how many I could stand but refused the painkiller pethidine, which was offered to me. Wisely or not, I wanted to experience natural childbirth! While all this was happening the doctor and midwife began to argue over whether or not I should have an episiotomy. It all became a little heated until Louis and I (somewhat breathlessly) insisted I didn't want one! The body has an amazing capacity for working with pain, as I found out as I worked with it to help me cope better. Sitting up on the bed to give birth was impossible for me so, with Louis holding on to the bed sheet that I was grasping as I squatted on a floor mattress, I finally gave birth to a purple and grey baby girl. She weighed five pounds thirteen and a half ounces, a good weight I was told for a premature baby. All had gone smoothly until it was found that I had a retained placenta so, without delay, I was whisked off to the operating theatre to have it removed. I remember waking up with a dreadful headache and a sore throat, I assume from the breathing tubes, but the joy of having a healthy baby made the pain seem quite insignificant.

An anxious time ensued when it was confirmed that baby had jaundice and, what with varying hormone levels and the shock of seeing her lying in an incubator wearing nothing but felt goggles, I broke down. She was taken to the special care unit and lay under blue lights with feeding tubes down her tiny nose. The staff in the unit were incredibly caring and skilled so that very soon she was back under white lights. The next day she was out of the lights and back in the ward with me. By this time I was bottle feeding her as I was not producing breast milk. As I write this chapter, Esther is now a healthy thirty-three year old and expecting her first baby around the same date that she was due!

My stay at King's stretched out to nine days during which time little Esther was given excellent care and attention. We were so unprepared when she decided to arrive but Louis and my mother now had plenty of time to purchase necessary items such as nappy buckets, a baby bath and a pram, while my father kindly finished decorating the nursery, a lovely little room at the back of our terraced house.

Shortly after giving birth I saw Dr L for a check-up and all seemed well. In his letter to my GP dated 8 November, he wrote:

> Marilyn had of course failed to breastfeed which was
> not surprising since she had very low prolactin levels
> in association with her hypopituitarism.

I also saw Mr W on 14 November whose first comment was that he remembered me from the previous year when I came to him 'in a terrible mess'. He pronounced me fit and asked me to start taking oestrogen (Harmogen tablets) straight away and progesterone (Provera tablets) on 1 December. Esther continued to thrive and we delighted in watching the changes taking place with each day.

Time flew by as we watched our lovely daughter developing and it wasn't long before we realised we would soon need a larger home. Within only a couple of weeks we found one and at the end of June 1984 moved into a house a short distance away. For quite a few days after settling in it felt as though we were on holiday and that eventually we would have to return to our tiny terraced house! That autumn I enrolled for drawing and yoga classes. Esther was happy to be looked after in the crèche while I had some time to myself. I had also returned to school, teaching only one day a week. It was good to keep my hand in as it were and it also gave my mother the opportunity to spend time with her granddaughter. I considered myself very lucky to have such a wonderful, supportive mum who was always happy and willing to share a day each week with Esther.

A few months into 1985 Louis and I decided the time was right to plan for a little sibling for Esther and on 8 May, I attended the infertility clinic at King's once again for an injection of Pergonal. Dr S had left the clinic by now but I was under the care of a friendly and efficient lady doctor. Ah, I thought, here we go again, another life, more sleepless nights, more pain but also more joy and love. I had a second injection on the 10 May. By 13 May my follicle had grown to 11 mm and I was told I may be ready for the booster injection (HCG) the following week. By the third visit my follicle was 14 mm but not quite ready. On the 17 May it was shown to have grown to more than 18 mm so I was given the booster injection. I've noted that on the 26 May I was aware of a knotty sensation below my tummy button. I'd had the same feeling after I conceived with Esther but I did not dare to presume anything! It was clear however that I was experiencing other signs of early pregnancy so wasn't surprised when, on 14 June, my scan revealed that, after only one cycle of treatment, I was pregnant and could expect to give birth around 7 February 1986. The doctor jokingly remarked that if I did not have a pituitary problem I may have had trouble not getting pregnant! Again, I was very happy and so was everyone else.

Before ever proceeding with Pergonal I was warned that treatment with this fertility drug can result in multiple births. This wasn't an issue the first time around. However, this time the doctor could see from the scan what she thought looked like a younger embryo lying with the established one, which clearly had a heartbeat. I can still hear her words, 'How do you feel about having twins?' then in an almost reassuring tone telling me the younger embryo could be an empty follicle or sac. I would have to wait another two weeks before she could be sure. It wasn't until I got home that the possibility of having twins hit me. Could I cope? Then I told myself not to be so silly, knowing that so many parents do cope. The next two weeks seemed to pass incredibly slowly and each day I wondered what the outcome would be.

It was time to return to the clinic for my scan. I still remember experiencing a surprising sense of loss on being told I was going to have one baby and not two. Thankfully, this sad feeling didn't last too long as I realised a healthy embryo was developing normally and already moving its little arms about. The empty sac had been reabsorbed into the bloodstream.

At the end of July I saw Dr L who was pleased with my news and said he wanted to keep in touch throughout the pregnancy. He thought I would need more oestrogen after the baby was born as my hair had been very fine before I became pregnant. It was a real luxury to have thicker, healthier hair during my pregnancies and I knew I would miss it after giving birth. I was thirsty again, but this time I craved a healthier option than during my previous pregnancy in the form of fizzy water – and possibly kept a certain natural mineral water company in business!

The next scan of baby 'Sam' or 'Rachel' was on 10 September and there he or she was, moving around quite happily, clenching and unclenching tiny fingers and kicking sturdy feet. Visits to the antenatal clinic confirmed that all was progressing as expected. In the meantime, as my size increased, so did Esther's curiosity! There was a lot going on in our lives: meeting friends with their children, the local mother and toddler group, swimming lessons, outings with nanna, and I continued with gentle yoga and painting classes. By mid-November I was getting very little sleep at night thanks to heartburn and had to prop myself up with multiple pillows, which helped a little. Eventually my GP decided to prescribe a mild sedative which worked but left me feeling quite hung over the next day. In December the situation improved and on 11 December I visited the antenatal clinic where I was very happy to be informed that baby was head down, almost ready to go!

Christmas was on the horizon and with it much excitement but this didn't stop poor Esther contracting a very nasty tummy bug which necessitated visits from our GP. Thankfully, she recovered after a few days but then, on Christmas Eve, I knew I had caught it. I was so ill the doctor came and gave me a 100 mg hydrocortisone injection as I couldn't keep anything down. Things weren't a great deal better the next day and I clearly remember my wonderful GP sitting on the floor in our hallway saying 'But why don't you want to go into hospital, Marilyn?', 'Because it's Christmas Day,' I weakly responded. Of course he was right. It was possible I would need extra hydrocortisone injections and, very importantly, baby needed to be monitored. The staff at King's tried their best to make the time a festive one, for all the patients. I was confined to a room but allowed to join the 'festivities' on Boxing Day although I found it difficult to eat anything. The main thing was that baby was safe and well. It was so good to be back home on 28 December and Louis and I even managed a couple of hours at a neighbour's New Year's Eve party.

My diary entry for 14 January reads, 'I'm enormous and look like a house end. More Braxton Hicks contractions today.' These continued regularly but when I visited the antenatal clinic on 29 January I was told they were B waves (stronger and longer than Braxton Hicks). The baby's due date of 7 February was drawing very close. This baby was obviously not in the same hurry as her sister had been but after an examination at the clinic on 5 February, contractions began. Snow fell as I kissed Esther goodnight. Louis and I left her in the safe care of my mother and drove off to King's.

No two pregnancies or deliveries are the same. This time my waters would not break so we waited and waited, but as time went on and on the doctor and midwife decided they had to break them for me. Once the floodgates opened an astonished doctor looked on in amazement at the amount of water gushing forth! As the contractions deepened in intensity, I decided to accept gas and air but found it didn't alleviate the pain much at all so finally threw the mask onto the floor and got on with yelling and pushing. Again, sitting on a bed was not an option for me so, with Louis supporting me under one arm and a midwife under the other, I experienced the thrill and relief of giving birth to Rachel – a second beautiful daughter. Later, Dr L came to see me to check that all was well with my levels of hydrocortisone following my injection of 100 mg before the delivery. All had gone smoothly so it was good to hear that, only two days after Rachel's birth, we could go home.

As we left the warm, security of the hospital, I was reminded of William Blake's poem *Infant Sorrow*. Despite its grittiness it never fails to make me smile:

> My mother groaned! My father wept.
> Into the dangerous world I leapt:
> Helpless, naked, piping loud;
> Like a fiend hid in a cloud.
>
> Struggling in my father's hands:
> Striving against my swaddling bands:
> Bound and weary I thought best
> To sulk upon my mother's breast.

3

Getting it right!

How much hydrocortisone to take and when

Poison is in everything, and no thing is without poison.
The dosage makes it either a poison or a remedy.

Paracelsus

As snow fell on 6 February 1986, Rachel entered a busier world than her sister had in 1983. Many established routine events were going on but she very quickly adapted to the noise of little people and adults as our social whirl continued, very often responding with wide smiles. I was soon able to resume art and yoga classes but also attended King's for regular checks. Mr W continued to monitor my oestrogen and progesterone and Dr L my hydrocortisone and thyroxine. In June he proposed that I spend a day in hospital to have a glucagon tolerance test to assess my cortisone levels.

For this test I was injected with glucagon – a hormone that works to raise blood sugar levels – and blood was taken every half hour. I remember feeling strange and quite weak afterwards as I'd had to stop taking hydrocortisone before the procedure. Half way through the test, Dr L brought his students along to let them see this strange lady with her rare condition. While the students looked on, Dr L referred to my 'Pond's' complexion and its cause, which he thought, was due to stunted release of the growth hormone. And I thought I'd inherited it from my mother who had perfect skin! (Interestingly, nothing was said at the time about growth hormone replacement but I have recently learned from my endocrinologist that growth hormone replacement was not around then, only being introduced in the late 1980s).

It had amused and intrigued me to be told during my consultation in June that my case was too complicated and rare to give to a medical student to study as a case history. It made me wonder if sufficient time is indeed given to students to study endocrinology, especially as my very efficient GP acknowledged that he didn't know enough about pituitary conditions. In an issue of Pituitary Life[3] entitled *The Pituitary and the GP*, I learned that medical students are attached to various consultants during their medical training, including endocrinologists but that, despite much learning activity, 'there is a low chance of close involvement with pituitary patients for the majority of students, unless one of their attachments was with a consultant endocrinologist'. The article goes on to say that even then, 'most of their work would be with diabetes...'. It is understandable that, as the symptoms of pituitary disease are extremely varied and similar to those of other diseases, misdiagnosis can be made (as I found out many years ago). In addition, 'only a tiny proportion of people with these symptoms will turn out to have pituitary disease'. My GP told me that I was the only pituitary patient on the practice records and this is borne out by the author's comment that 'Most GPs could expect to be involved in the diagnosis of one new pituitary patient in their career, compared with hundreds of other conditions...'. In the six years since this article was written it may be that the recommendations given in the article have been followed through and that more GPs are aware that they need to look for other signs and symptoms and arrange for more specific tests and/or referrals. The author also cites the case of a pituitary diagnosis discovered through an optician's report which described partial loss of vision which, he explains, 'is typical of pituitary enlargement'. At the time of writing, I have received a poster which I requested from The Pituitary Foundation to give to my optician in the hope that it will draw their attention to the fact that visual field tests can detect pituitary tumours. The Foundation produces a range of Awareness leaflets for GPs too and these, together with access to their website, provide all doctors with information they need.

Now, back to the glucagon test! The following extract from Dr L's letter to my GP dated 17 July 1986 gives the following results:

> This [test] had been done because this patient's base line cortisols had been <30 nmol/1. Indeed during the glucagon tolerance test her cortisols remained at this level confirming that she had severe secondary adrenal insufficiency. This test had been carried out because of a variety of symptoms which she had experienced when changing the dose of hydrocortisone. This result indicates that she therefore needs to double the dose of hydrocortisone whenever she feels unwell, as she has no underlying adrenal reserve to mount her own response to supplement her maintenance dose. She is to continue taking hydrocortisone 20 mg in the morning and 10 mg in the evening and thyroxine 150 micrograms daily.

Today, the normal dose for hydrocortisone is 15–20 mg split over two or three times a day. I have often asked myself why my dose is higher than this. Was I given too high a dose when I was first diagnosed with hypopituitarism? I asked my endocrinologist about this recently and he told me that less hydrocortisone is given now as more research shows evidence that people don't produce as much of this hormone as was thought. The change is not huge however and in terms of bone density it can have made a little difference but not as much as massive doses would have, say in cases when steroids are given to treat a severe illness, so it is important to distinguish between the two situations. This is reassuring but there is still a niggling concern at the back of my mind about the little difference a higher dose could have made over the years.

Every endocrinologist I have seen has explained when and why it is necessary to increase my hydrocortisone intake. I've learned about how the body responds to stress caused by illness or shock when the adrenals naturally increase the levels of cortisol required. With pituitary patients, it is essential to increase the dose of hydrocortisone to imitate, as far as possible, the body's natural response. The normal system of both adults and children has a circadian rhythm which peaks to meet stressful situations, indicating that the adrenals are responding to the body's needs. Production of cortisol starts to steadily increase around 2am, peaking at around 6.30am, which is why it is important for me to take my first hydrocortisone dose upon waking. I know that if I don't take it before I get out of bed, I begin to feel light-headed very quickly! I was taking my second dose around 5pm by which time my body was telling me it needed it! This was the regime I was advised to follow when diagnosed in 1982 but recently I have been told by my endocrine nurse and endocrinologist that I can split my dose by taking 15 mg in the morning, 10 mg at midday and 5 mg in the evening. I have tried this and found that I don't feel so tired in the afternoons, which is great.

The time in which a dose of hydrocortisone is absorbed varies in different people so it is important that it is tailored to the individual. In an interesting article in Pituitary Life[4], the author explains that one of the more common symptoms experienced by hypopituitary patients is tiredness, fatigue and sometimes exhaustion. She clearly explains that:

> Circadian rhythms are physical, mental and
> behavioural changes that follow a 24-hour cycle,
> responding primarily to light and darkness in a
> person's environment. These rhythms can change
> hormone release, body temperature and other
> important bodily functions.

The author recommends that hypopituitary patients take their replacement hormones to mimic the more natural rhythms. This makes sense, especially as:

> Cortisol, thyroxine and testosterone all have rhythms
> but we can't quite replicate the physiological levels
> with replacement hormones.

It turned out that taking my hydrocortisone three times a day, i.e. morning, midday and evening, better matched my body's natural release of cortisol. If you are a hypopituitary patient reading this who is taking Plenadren (modified release hydrocortisone) instead of hydrocortisone tablets, your regime will of course be different.

I always double my steroids to deal with infections and nasty viruses such as a tummy bug. Usually, I remain on this higher dose until the virus has gone then start to decrease until I reach my normal daily dose. This has to be done gradually to avoid feeling very odd, tired and as though I have a hangover! As I have learned to my cost, even too much time in the sunshine can cause a lot of stress on the body and I've had to respond quickly by doubling my dose. There have been times when I have needed to increase just a little to cope with everyday emotional, physical or mental stress such as situations at work or unexpected upsetting events when my body feels suddenly deprived of cortisol. Along with other excellent publications, The Pituitary Foundation has published a very helpful leaflet[5] giving advice for the pituitary patient taking hydrocortisone, including recommendations for changes in dose.

Sometimes doubling the dose of hydrocortisone with tablets isn't enough which is what happened before Rachel's arrival and over the years there have been three further incidents of food poisoning and gastric flu. On these occasions a doctor or nurse visited to administer the 100 mg dose except once, when Louis came to the rescue! This was possible as I always keep a supply of hydrocortisone sodium phosphate ampoules, syringes and needles at home in case of emergencies. My doctor has written a letter to show to airport, port or rail personnel if necessary, stating that I need to carry my medication, as well as needles and injectable preparations, with me whenever I travel. It makes sense to take them with me whenever I take trips in this country too. Hydrocortisone tablets are always tucked away safely in my handbag just in case I may need to increase my dose or when I know I'm going to be out and about when my midday or evening dose is due. This can be quite tricky at times and I've been known to dive behind displays in shops or grope around in my bag for my tablets on public transport! I feel safer carrying not just my tablets around with me but also a blue Steroid Treatment Card, MedicAlert card, and wearing a MedicAlert bracelet that gives details of my condition and informs medical personnel that I'm vulnerable to an adrenal crisis. It seems there is a lot to think about but it eventually becomes second nature and not such a stressful thing as it may be at first! But, of all the items I carry around with me, probably the most important is the London Ambulance Service NHS Trust Patient Specific Protocol for steroid dependent patients which I downloaded from The Pituitary Foundation website. This is to be shown to the ambulance crew immediately upon their arrival. It tells them to administer 100 mg of hydrocortisone in the event of a steroid dependent crisis. I have only needed to use it once and desperately hope I never need to use it again. The thought of experiencing another adrenal crisis remains my greatest fear but I intend to avoid it ever happening again, if possible.

That eventful day in September 2012 is etched in my memory, a day when the levels of cortisol in my blood became greatly reduced and this adrenal insufficiency led to an adrenal crisis, which is life threatening

It had started off cool and cloudy so I had dressed cautiously, expecting it to become much cooler. It didn't. Instead, as I walked along Oxford Street I found myself feeling more and more uncomfortable as the heat of the day increased. After stopping to have lunch and drinking at least two glassfuls of water with my meal, I began to feel better so carried on to do some shopping. It was hot and airless on the train home as the sun glared through the window, reminding me of the hot sunshine of the previous days when I had worn a sun hat, thinking that I was well protected. Once home I rested, noticing that I was feeling tired and a little light-headed but put this down to the heat and activities of the day. After an early dinner I drove to a friend's house for one of our regular get-togethers and looked forward to chatting and catching up with our news. Another friend joined us and soon the conversation took off but after about an hour I began to feel a strong, deep pain in my stomach. This can indicate the need for more hydrocortisone so I took an extra 10 mg tablet. I was sure this would ease the problem but when there were no signs of any change I instinctively told my friends I would have to leave. As I drove the fifteen minute journey home I knew I was experiencing something quite different and that it was serious. I drove on, knowing that if I stopped to take more tablets I would have had no one to help me and I dreaded the thought of having to use my mobile phone to call for help while I was alone. Willpower is an amazing thing and I used this to continue driving and to will the traffic lights ahead to turn green. Thankfully, they did and there ahead of me at last was the road where I live. As I stopped outside our house I noticed my heart was pounding as my breathing increased.

'Louis, get my hydrocortisone tablets, quick!' I called out as I stumbled through the door. Thank goodness he was home. He handed me the tablets and I took 30 mg as I sat down like a lump of lead at the kitchen table. Then, the convulsions began. Louis told me later, when he could think clearly, that he was afraid to leave me for a second let alone try to inject me with hydrocortisone. It was very obvious by now that I was experiencing something quite new and extremely frightening, an extreme situation which had come on quite suddenly and required professional help. I felt quite out of control yet managed to realise this must be an adrenal crisis and urged Louis to call an ambulance. He called and explained the situation and requested them to respond immediately, which they said they would. In the meantime I had staggered to the kitchen sink where I proceeded to vomit while my body shook with each convulsion. This prompted Louis to telephone 999 a second time describing what had happened. The person he spoke to said he would stay on the line until help arrived. By the time the first responder arrived I had collapsed onto the floor but somehow managed to form words begging the paramedic to inject me with 100 mg of hydrocortisone. It was hard to take in his response that I should have an injection of 200 mg instead and it was then that I remembered the Ambulance Protocol which, in my confused state, I had temporarily forgotten was in my handbag. As Louis retrieved it and handed it to him it was hard to believe what we heard. Paramedics do a wonderful job but what happened next could have had disastrous consequences as he reacted by telling us he had forgotten his reading glasses and couldn't see the instructions! Imagine the scene: A writhing, vomiting body on the floor, a perplexed yet amazingly calm husband and a confused and embarrassed paramedic. The stuff black comedies are made of.

Saved by the bell! An ambulance had pulled up outside and two paramedics walked in, read the protocol, which Louis had thrust into the hands of one of them, and immediately agreed I needed 100 mg of hydrocortisone. At last the first responder proceeded to inject this into my thigh. Within a fairly short space of time the convulsions and vomiting eased and I realised I was not dying!

As soon as I was able to get up off the floor I was helped into the ambulance outside and once again found myself on my way to King's College Hospital where I was put on a saline drip in the Accident & Emergency department and eventually seen by a doctor. Hours seemed to pass as the drip emptied its contents into my arm and I began to feel better. Perhaps I should have spent the night in hospital, as recommended by the doctor, but I would have waited some time before a bed was available. So, when given the option to go home, I grasped the opportunity to get back to the comfort of my own bed. Exhausted and desperate for sleep, several hours passed before I awoke. I took 90 mg of hydrocortisone that day then gradually reduced my dose.

The causes of adrenal insufficiency are varied. They include illness, emotional stress and being under medicated. My endocrinologist believed dehydration had triggered the adrenal crisis that day and, although I thought I had consumed an adequate amount of water, maybe I had not had enough in my system to counter the effects of quite a lot of heat and sunshine. It is unfortunate that I've had to experience such a terrifying event to become fully aware of the causes and effects of an adrenal crisis. I'm very aware now, as are my family and close friends, who I know will come to my rescue should it happen again, although I would dearly love to spare them the experience.

My experience induced fear, vulnerability, and anxiety. Realising that an adrenal crisis is life threatening, part of me reluctantly remains apprehensive about even the slightest possibility that a very small minority of health professionals may not react with the speed and skill required to avert a coma, or worse. However, I tell myself that I am well prepared and equipped for it not to happen again. I am determined to be positive and embrace life as I look forward to continuing to do the things I am still capable of doing without any such fear getting in the way!

4

Time moves on

Time is a great teacher, but unfortunately it kills all its pupils

Hector Louis Berlioz

So back now to January 1987, on a day when an eight inch blanket of snow covers the road and pavement outside. The temperature drops to five degrees below freezing, taking me back to my winters in Toronto in the late 1960s, although they were even colder. Attempts to take the children out fail miserably, as pushchair wheels stubbornly grind to a halt. In the loft, the water tank freezes but, upon a neighbour's advice, I open the hatch and, as the warm air slowly rises, the ice gradually melts sending water gushing through taps once again. Louis is away on business and I'm grateful for the action of kind neighbours who come to the rescue with food and essentials. Then my mother rings to say she has slipped in a puddle of rain water on her landing, blown in through an open window by the freezing wind, and broken her wrist. Quite a start to the year!

February brought brighter, milder weather and a visit to King's. Dr L had explained that a colleague was interested in taking a blood sample from me for analysis following a recent discovery that animals with low prolactin levels have an inefficient immune system and they were interested to see if humans are similarly affected. I was glad to help and didn't mind being a guinea pig, especially as my immune system didn't seem to be wonderfully efficient. However, it wasn't until June that I was asked to attend the hospital to give the blood sample, and I had to wait until February 1988 before I was told that there wasn't enough scientific evidence to show that prolactin levels affect the immune system. Oh well, it was worth a try!

By September, I found myself in the classroom once again, after being asked to work one day a week in a different inner London primary school. This would be just right, I thought, and would give my mother the chance to have Esther and Rachel all to herself every Thursday. I was so fortunate to have her support and the girls were excited to be having a 'nanna day' every week. Of course there were times when I wondered whether I should have made this commitment, especially on days when I had to drag myself in after a disturbed night!

Some readers may remember the reassuring words of Michael Fish when he gave the weather forecast on the evening of 15 October 1987, telling us that we weren't going to be visited by a hurricane. At the same time, Louis rang from Brittany to say they were experiencing gale force winds and, when I was awoken in the middle of the night by the battering of those well-travelled winds against the bedroom window pane, I knew something wasn't quite right. History was made when, for the first time in 300 years, winds reaching 100 mph hit London and the south. We awoke to the sad sight of a number of trees which, despite their former seeming invincibility, now lay uprooted across the road outside. Garden fences also lay flat on the ground and roof tiles sat heavily on lawns and pavements. The recovery process was long and arduous.

By 1988 life was certainly busy but fulfilling, despite occasions when I felt exhausted. I think it was in May when I spoke to my GP about episodes of being 'wiped out' and having strange muscular sensations and he told me to increase my hydrocortisone and make an appointment to see my endocrinologist. Dr L agreed that if I felt better on a higher dose then to continue with this! I did but only for a short time, knowing that high doses of hydrocortisone can affect the immune system. My next visit to see Dr L in June found me facing a very tired doctor after I'd had to wait for two hours with two small children, who had behaved extremely well considering how boring it must have been for them. It was a routine check but when I asked about the results of a blood test I'd had on the previous visit, he gave me the unexpected reply, 'What blood test?' He then proceeded to demonstrate how his new blood pressure machine worked! I remember feeling quite low as I left, wondering what I had gained from my visit.

When I caught a nasty 'flu virus in July, Louis took matters into his own hands, particularly when I told him about the doctor's remark about the blood test. He contacted the private health company he was insured with through his company and arranged for me to see an endocrinologist in the private sector. It was time for a second opinion and, hopefully, to discover why I was catching so many viruses and whether these occurrences had any relationship to my condition. I must say, I wasn't too keen on the idea initially as it seemed to go against my principles.

I attended London Bridge Hospital for my private appointment with Dr N later that month. Immediately, I felt I had been transported to another age with friendly nurses gliding casually around the clinic in-between directing patients to the coffee machine and taking blood samples. The doctor had one hour of uninterrupted time to give me when many revelations were made. Only a few days after my appointment I returned for my test results. I left feeling quite emotional, a little angry and amazed. It turned out that my thyroxine levels had been too high (although not dangerously so) which, I was told, creates the need for more cortisol, resulting in my body being in a state of chemical imbalance.

Indeed, replacement medication may affect other hormone levels, as examined in a 2013 edition of *Pituitary Life*.[6] The authors state that 'replacement therapy of multiple hormones in pituitary diseases is complex'. They look at the hormones used in pituitary diseases and the interactions between them. I will simply refer to the interaction between cortisol and thyroxine replacement as this is most relevant here. The authors state that, 'replacement doses of hydrocortisone are unlikely to affect the thyroid hormones and the levothyroxine replacement dose' (T4 in tablet form, which I had been prescribed) but stress that an evaluation of the cortisol levels is mandatory before starting thyroid hormone replacement to avoid a steroid crisis in patients with untreated adrenal insufficiency.

In another article in the October 2011 issue of *Pituitary Life*,[7] the author explains that doctors can have difficulty interpreting thyroid blood tests in patients with pituitary disease, especially if they are not specialists in endocrinology. It can be difficult for doctors to know exactly what free T4 level to aim for when starting a patient off on levothyroxine ('free T4' and 'free T3' are thyroid hormones in the blood controlled by levels of TSH, or thyroid-stimulating hormone). In the study carried out it was discovered that some patients with pituitary disease were not being given enough levothyroxine to keep free T4 levels 'up to the range which we know represents optimal replacement in people with a normal pituitary'. With too little thyroid hormone in the body, everything slows with the patient experiencing, for example, tiredness, dry skin and slowness in thinking, all of which I experienced before treatment. On the other hand, too much thyroid replacement can cause everything to speed up with the increased risk of heart rhythm problems. Whenever he examined me, Dr N asked if I had palpitations so he must have been checking to see whether I was receiving too much levothyroxine.

I wondered why my thyroxine levels had not been checked since 1982 when I was prescribed 150 mcg (micrograms) of thyroxine daily or whether this could have been explained by the missing blood test mentioned earlier. Dr N adjusted my thyroxine intake to 150 mcg/100 mcg on alternate days and I was told I needed to have blood tests every six months. He also gave me a list of advisory notes regarding how to respond to illnesses and recommended that I should join the Pituitary Foundation. A blood test result in September showed that my thyroxine levels were now normal. I also felt much more confident about when to increase my hydrocortisone. During a routine visit to see my GP a few weeks later, he agreed with me that it was regrettable that I'd had to go to the private sector to discover all of this.

I seemed to experience quite a few episodes of viral infections. On one occasion when I telephoned Dr N for advice about whether or not I was taking enough hydrocortisone to deal with a current infection, he recommended I double my dose for at least five days before reducing it very gradually to avoid feeling extremely tired and disorientated. Decreasing had to be done in tiny amounts – 5 mg every three days. He also suggested that I took this higher dose three times a day to mimic my body rhythms and to start a course of antibiotics. Dr N was helpful in giving me a four week regime for 'coming down' to allow my body to get used to each lower stage. As soon as I got back to my normal daily dose, I felt my energy returning. Dr N also gave me a blood pressure kit – the old fashioned type – which Louis attempted to use on me, nearly costing me an arm!

The months flew by. By 1989 I was teaching at a local school for two days a week. Rachel spent one of those days with my mother and on the other day she enjoyed going to playgroup and then to a friend's house. By this time, Esther was at full-time nursery. My school was only a five minute walk from where they spent their days so very convenient for us all. I had also re-joined a yoga class, stretching parts of me I had forgotten existed. Around this time, Dr N altered my thyroxine intake to 100 mcg on day one, 100 mcg on day two and 150 mcg on the third day. This could be a little confusing but I somehow managed the new regime! I also saw Mr W who was pleased with my progress but told me that when I reached 50 years of age I should have a bone density scan to see how much oestrogen, if any, I would need to continue to take. I record on 17 June how thrilled I was to feel so much better and was sure this was due to having my hormone levels balanced. By October, however, after much frustration involving builders working on our kitchen extension, which seemed to take forever (we were promised a new kitchen by Christmas and I should have asked 'Which Christmas?'), I woke with an upset stomach and aching joints. Dr N advised me over the telephone to double my hydrocortisone. My blood pressure was low and would have been lower if I hadn't increased. Oh, the joys of the effects of stress!

In May 1989, the headteacher of the primary school where I had been working on a part-time basis, offered me a full-time post. I was excited by the prospects and was sure I could do it as Esther and Rachel were now in full-time education. A wonderful neighbour, who had children of her own, offered to take the girls to school, collect them then bring them to me in my classroom in the afternoons. This turned out to be the highlight of my day. Both girls were very happy with this arrangement as they had such fun in the company of my neighbour's children.

Just to put things into context, close to the end of the year, a significant event took place when the Berlin Wall was finally knocked down; then, in February 1990, Nelson Mandela was released from prison after twenty-seven years, his release triggering relaxation, at last, of apartheid laws in South Africa.

During the summer of 1990 I visited King's menopause clinic and this time saw a different doctor. She explained that many of the symptoms I was now experiencing, such as shoulder stiffness, tiredness, dry eyes and joint aches, could be due to lack of oestrogen. She decided to change my dose and told me I would now be taking Premarin, about which I felt quite uncomfortable as it is collected from the urine of pregnant mares. She also changed my progesterone tablets. A few days later I felt terribly tired, my shoulders were stiff and my joints ached, but after taking an extra tablet the symptoms began to ease.

Unfortunately, some of the symptoms persisted and in April 1991 the doctor increased my oestrogen and decreased my progesterone. By August I was feeling at my best. All my hormone replacement seemed at last to be balanced. Despite the problems related to getting this particular hormone balance right, I enjoyed my work, even taking on a language post and beginning to write the school language policy. Family and friends were marvellous and always supported me, although one or two thought I was mad! But perhaps they were right as the stress involved left me feeling shattered at times and, rather than stop for a few days' rest, I would occasionally increase my hydrocortisone to get me through events and commitments. This is not something I would do now! There were, of course, days when I had to give in and take to my bed, especially when the dreaded 'flu struck. During one particularly nasty outbreak I remember all the teachers around me seemed to be collapsing in a heap and these were healthy people with normal pituitary function. It was the year the National Curriculum SATS (Standard Assessment Tests) were introduced and, as I was teaching a Year 2 class, I was responsible for preparing and testing children I already knew well enough to 'test' without a government directive! The pressure was on myself, the class and in fact the entire school. Drama and art had to be curtailed as I focussed on testing over a period of weeks. Some children enjoyed the challenge whereas one or two found it just too much and, no matter how much I reassured them, cried when presented with a task. In subsequent years it bothered me to have to tick boxes as a form of measuring achievement and although standards needed to improve, for me the heart seemed to have gone out of teaching, reducing spontaneity and development of the whole child.

I sometimes wonder when I found the time to write anything in my diary but somehow I managed to record not only hospital visits, but events with family and friends. Time marched on, but by the end of 1993 and after another bout of 'flu which left me completely drained, I reluctantly took the decision to approach the headteacher of my school and tell her of my decision to reduce my teaching hours. It was time to be kinder to my body.

5

Things start to change

Progress is impossible without change ...
George Bernard Shaw

The board of governors of my school finally agreed that, from January 1994, I could work three days a week, with a job-share partner covering the remaining two days. The pressure was off a little and I looked forward to having time to breathe.

Two significant events occurred in May that year. Nelson Mandela was elected President of South Africa and the Channel Tunnel was opened, connecting Britain with our neighbour, France. A time to be optimistic about the future. Upon hearing the news about the opening of the Channel Tunnel, I was swiftly taken back in time to the early 1970s when I was employed by management consultants who were working on the cost– benefit study for the then proposed building of a tunnel under the Channel. I must have typed a number of telephone directory-sized reports, sometimes working at weekends, to complete them before the deadline. As we all know, that proposal was abandoned due to economic reasons, but now it was really happening!

In that same month a much less dramatic event occurred – I attended Guy's hospital in London for my first bone density test. It was straightforward. I just had to lie under a moving scanner as it took pictures of my spine and femur. The results showed that, although my bone density measurements were just below average, they were well within the normal range. I was to have a further test in about eighteen months' time.

Then, in July, I somehow managed to damage a tendon in my

right arm. This coincided with my decision to leave my primary school to take a break from teaching for however long I needed. I remember saying an emotional goodbye to everyone there, children, parents and staff, and it left me pondering what to do next. I carried on writing notes in my diary using my left hand so the result was a spider's scrawl of very basic information. This called for an increase of 10 mg of hydrocortisone for a while to help deal with the pain and which my GP recommended. It was frustrating not being able to write with my right hand (physiotherapist's orders) or play the piano, although I managed to drive short distances. My neck was also affected so I occasionally wore a collar. Dr N ordered a neck X-ray which my records state revealed:

> ... severe degeneration disease between C5 and C7
> with some osteophytic encroachment on the exit
> foramina on the left side.

I understand this to mean that degeneration in the spinal column had caused an obstruction in the open space on the left side of the vertebrae through which the spinal nerve passes, causing pressure on the nerve, resulting in both local and referred pain. His comment, 'You have the neck of an 82 year old woman,' didn't help my morale! All this began in August and by November Dr N explained to me that a further X-ray showed more degeneration of the discs in my lumbar region. I was now experiencing pain in my right thigh which turned out to be a trapped sciatic nerve.

By December I was finding it very hard to sit anywhere, although the pain in my arm had improved somewhat and I could write a little better. Lying down in bed was not comfortable so I took to sleeping on the floor, wrapping myself in duvets. Surprisingly, this was quite cosy and less painful! A further X-ray showed that my lumbar seemed okay but that I had osteoarthritis in my hips. Dr N believed this problem was related to my hypopituitarism.

It seemed that, out of the blue, my entire body was reacting to something. Burning pain persisted in my upper arms, occasionally moving to my lower arms. I had some stiffness in my hip joints and sometimes severe pain across my right thigh. A scan of my lower back showed, thankfully, that the discs were not degenerating and Dr N now thought that I was suffering from osteoarthritis in my hip joints. Gradually, the pain in my arms became less severe but I was unable to raise them for some time so at yoga, when everyone else stretched their arms out in perfect alignment, mine were at half-mast! I wondered what was happening to me as my leg and hip joints remained stiff and I was finding that even short walks to the local shops produced aching and stiffness.

By January 1995 the pain in my arms was becoming less frequent but my hips and right thigh continued to ache and seize up when I sat for too long. Physiotherapy helped, as well as some hydrotherapy, and although yoga helped too, I needed to rest afterwards. I was referred by Dr N to a neurologist who didn't think that my thigh pain was a nerve problem but that instead it was emanating from my hip. I record that, since my physical problems presented themselves, I had not liked the resulting inactivity but I unwillingly accepted the situation, longing for it to end! The next time I spoke to Dr N he suggested that my leg problem was caused by calcium crystals deposited on the muscle tendons attached to the femur and that osteoarthritis was not really the problem after all. 'I don't know whether I'm coming or going,' I wrote in my diary that day. According to Dr N, both my leg and neck problems had developed because of my pituitary condition. He believed this was the case because my body had not been receiving normal levels of hormones before I was diagnosed and treated.

February arrived and with it a box of books presented to me at the door by a very disgruntled looking postman. Open University books. I had decided that, to save my sanity now that I was not working and to distract me from what was going on with my body, I would study for an Advanced Diploma in Special Educational Needs, taking the Foundation level in the first year. Having worked with many children experiencing special educational needs such as dyspraxia and dyslexia, I was interested in discovering more with a view to being able to meet their needs more effectively in the future, once I was fit again. It was time to put my brain into gear I thought, as I tackled my first assignment!

By this time I was able to hold my arms up during my yoga lessons, although only for a little while but at least this was an improvement. However, my right thigh and leg continued to trouble me, especially when attempting to get up from a sitting position. If a chair was too low or soft, the muscle in my right thigh seemed to 'lock' as I got up and it could take minutes of gentle manoeuvring before I could stand. It got to the point that, no matter where I went, I had to test chairs or benches to make sure they were comfortable. A bit like Goldilocks in the popular children's story. But strength was returning to my arms and the pain was less severe. My right leg was improving although I was still finding walking for more than fifteen minutes a bit of a problem. At a consultation with Dr N in March my blood pressure was found to be very low so it was suggested I raise my hydrocortisone 10 mg. This would also help deal with the pain in my hip and leg. Some days the leg pain behaved quite fiercely and I found myself having great difficulty getting up from a chair, still having to ease and twist very carefully as I did so. I became quite a contortionist! It made sense to drive to my Open University tutorials as walking and travelling on public transport was rather a challenge.

April arrived and with it a holiday in sunny Portugal. Soothing, healing sunshine and swimming in warm water, but not too much! By late May my arms gained even more strength although my back muscles 'burned' if I sat in one position for too long. Dr

N informed me that this was referred pain from the 4th and 5th vertebrae where X-rays showed the discs were partly worn. Apparently, the severe pain I experienced earlier was due to nerve entrapment in the 2nd and 3rd vertebrae where the discs had virtually disappeared. It was explained to me that the pain of this severe condition was improving as my brain began to recognise that the problem was associated with the lower discs, i.e. the burning sensation in my back and aching in my arms.

After some consideration, Dr N suggested that a cortisone injection into the muscle at the top of my right thigh should help alleviate the pain there. It had no effect. I must admit it was all becoming very confusing having been told so many different things over the past year. Dr N referred me to a rheumatologist but, on examination, he admitted I was a puzzling case! He diagnosed fibromyalgia, which, according to Dr N, is a diagnosis given when doctors don't know what is wrong with a patient! My legs continued to ache and burn and at times I felt extremely low and frustrated. Thank goodness I had my family, friends and my studies to distract me and cheer me up. The rheumatologist referred me to a physiotherapist he highly recommended. After she had pummelled me around a lot I seemed to experience some freedom of movement in my arms and by the end of July I reported that I could sit in one position for longer periods of time and felt strength returning to my legs. The only thing that hadn't changed was the sharp pain in my right thigh.

October, and exam time. How was I going to sit through two three-hour exams, despite some improvement in my back? I was still experiencing the odd 'seizing up' of my muscles there. The answer was physiotherapy before and after the exams! And I passed!

The year came to a close with a visit to King's menopause clinic once more where I had blood taken to test for oestrogen levels, the result of which showed excellent absorption. It had not been an easy year but I was grateful that it ended with some easement of the pain in my back and legs, despite the continuation of a sharp pain in my right thigh although this was not travelling so far. In preparation for my next year of study with the Open University I had arranged to teach on a voluntary basis at a local school for only two hours each week, starting in the New Year.

By then greater mobility was returning to my legs although I had to be careful not to overdo my walking to avoid the pain returning. Very early in the year Dr N told me he thought my problems mainly stemmed from wear and tear in my spine, or spondylosis, which was also affecting the muscles and nerves of my lumbar region. I was also continuing to experience a burning sensation in the muscles of my back and neck which worsened if I sat too long. Curiously, the pain in my leg muscles shifted to the top of my legs, which I noticed particularly if I sat still for too long, or walked for more than half an hour. I needed to be careful not to sit too long at the computer as I tried to complete my Open University assignments! Mentally, it was good for me to be working and studying, although I realised I was probably pushing myself physically. On the other hand I had to remember that I could not have taken on any work of this kind during the previous year which told me that, although the process was slow, my condition was improving. What I did notice was that I was more aware of the muscular pain when my hydrocortisone requirement increased. There were occasions when I felt extremely low and wondered when the problem would lift, then I'd feel guilty about this, remembering those in far worse situations. On 30 January 1996 I had my second bone density scan which showed below average results with the lumbar spine and femoral neck below the mean for my age but, compared to the previous scan in 1994, the femoral neck had not changed significantly and there had been a slight improvement in the lumbar spine measurement.

At this time I was offered a teaching post at yet another primary school, working only four hours a week with special needs children. I appreciated this as it would help towards my work with the Open University and wouldn't take up too much of my week. Despite many positive things going on in my life, I was struggling a little to come to terms with what was happening to my body and mentioned my partial anger about this to my GP. He recommended that I should have a few sessions with the Practice's counsellor. The first session left me feeling quite emotionally exhausted but further sessions proved to be quite cathartic in helping provide reasons for the physical changes and pain I was experiencing. Also, many thoughts and images combined to make some things clearer; for example, my need to be in control, my purpose in life and ways of contributing to it, as well as some personal issues. At the end of the course the excellent counsellor asked me to choose, from a number of picture postcards, an image that had special meaning to me. I chose one which showed a path stretching out towards light on the horizon. Symbolically, the end of the path would be the end of the pain. I marked where I was at that moment in time, which was roughly half way. With determination and effort I would one day reach the end of the path!

In the meantime, Dr N had prescribed various medications to reduce the pain, one of which was Molipaxin which he described as an antidepressant, assuring me that it was being prescribed because it acted like a steroid and should reduce the pain I was experiencing and enable me to sleep better. I must say I slept better but as I almost fell over in the middle of the night on one occasion when I needed to get up, I decided to reduce the dose. Eventually I stopped taking anything stronger than a paracetamol.

It's interesting how people come along at the right moment and offer help or point you in the right direction. A new gym had opened locally and I was guided towards it by a lady who had found the workout she was doing there very helpful. After an initial interview with a trainer, a fitness programme was arranged which addressed my needs, although I was advised to pace myself carefully. The thing I liked most about this personal gym was that there was a warm pool where I could give myself some hydrotherapy. It was bliss, especially on days when I was in great pain or after a physiotherapy session. I attended the gym until it closed down but as the year progressed I had more good days than bad, resulting in greater energy. What it is to be almost free of pain! I was able to give more to my lovely family, my work and my studies and to enjoy more time out with friends. I still had some not so good days when I was aware that if I sat for too long in one place, such as on a car journey, then my back and leg muscles became more painful. The joint area at the top of each leg gave me most pain, stiffening up quite badly at times. Dr N repeated his earlier remark that I was more aware of the pain due to my pituitary problem and that, although I receive hormone replacement therapy, it is not as efficient as normal production of these hormones in dealing with the type of pain I was experiencing.

After a visit to King's in October I received a letter from the menopause clinic with encouraging news:

> ... your recent oestrogen level shows a level of 639
> which is almost exactly the level which we would aim
> to keep it in order to protect your bones. I would
> recommend you continue with your current HRT ...

My first diary entry for 1997 records that mentally I wanted to get on with my Open University study, if only my body would allow! Unfortunately, I had caught a nasty 'flu virus. Up went my hydrocortisone dose to deal with it but I was interested to learn from Dr N that stress caused by having 'flu causes 'flu-like symptoms itself, which is what I was experiencing. At last, by the end of the month, I was back to teaching my special needs children. They were a challenging bunch but the results were mainly encouraging and the expression on their faces when they achieved was a joy to behold.

As the year progressed my body reminded me daily of nerve pain or muscle aches but at least I was able to work and enjoy time with family and friends. However, I did take some time out in March with a three day visit to Oxford while my mother looked after the girls until Louis came home from work. It was actually more of a retreat than a visit as I spent my time reading, visiting galleries and museums, generally wandering around the town admiring the architecture and wallowing in the space I had to myself. I returned home a new woman! Yet by July my GP commented that it looked as though I was 'stuck' with fibromyalgia! I came to terms with it being a matter of time and patience before things improved. Near the end of the year a third bone density scan revealed no significant change since the previous scan in 1996.

Nineteen ninety-eight arrived, the year when I, together with close friends, reached our half century. I began a new teaching post, this time working with bi-lingual pupils. I was also in the final year of my Open University course which, if I passed, would mean having achieved a Master's degree in Education which incorporated an Advanced Diploma in Special Educational Needs. What I would do with it I had no idea as I knew a full-time career in teaching was out of the question but I hoped it would prepare me for a part-time post where I could apply much of what I had learned to the job. By now I was only recording significant events in my diary but even these were concise.

Notes written in September record that my right leg and lower back continued to trouble me. Dr N referred me to another rheumatologist who sent me off for an MRI. This showed I had a disc prolapse and further investigations revealed degenerative disc disease in the lower three cervical segments with osteophyte encroachment at the exit foramine of C5–7 on the left side. Almost total fusion of the sacroiliac joints was revealed and degenerative changes at L5/S1. By October my perspective of the world changed as I spent much time viewing it from the floor. The pain was spiteful, aggressive, mocking and teasing as it eased then decided to bite back again. Physiotherapy sessions started and by the end of the month my sacrum area had relaxed but the pain caused by the protruding disc shown on the MRI still yelled and the sciatic nerve in my right leg continued to scream. It was impossible for me to work. My final exam with the Open University was due but they were so helpful in arranging special facilities at their Finchley site in north London and I remember sitting uncomfortably at a desk but able to get up and walk around whenever I needed to. Other students, apart from a very pregnant lady, appeared to have problems affecting their mobility. Friends called in regularly which was wonderful and always cheered me up as by now I was spending most of my time on the living room floor. Laughter – what a wonderful way to lose weight! Rather than coming to the rescue, anti-inflammatories only upset my system. In the meantime the pain seemed to enjoy moving around. 'It continues,' groaned Dr N on my next visit.

An X-ray in December showed inflammation in my right hip which seemed to be the cause of the problem in my leg. How pain dulls the senses, suffocates the creative mind, I wrote. Things seemed to drag on until, finally, the rheumatologist decided I needed a body scan. He telephoned me to report that this had revealed more than general wear and tear in my hip, something he was extremely angry about, remarking that the MRI technician should have noticed this. In other words, I needed to see an orthopaedic surgeon.

6

It goes on!

Surgeons can cut out everything except cause
Herbert M Shelton

I know that many people who do not have a pituitary condition suffer from osteoarthritis and osteoporosis and I cannot categorically state or prove that the effects on my bones are due to my pituitary condition. However, I do feel that a contributory factor must be not having a natural flow of hormones in my body for almost ten years of my life and lack of growth hormone for much longer than that. Over the years this has been corroborated by the comments of various doctors, endocrinologists and surgeons. So the rest of this story mainly focuses on the possible effects of those 'ten lost years'.

The day I had been waiting for with great anticipation, 4 January 1999, arrived at last and with it a mixture of hope and relief. As walking had now become extremely difficult, Louis and I drove to London Bridge Hospital where I hobbled into the consultation room to meet Mr N, the orthopaedic surgeon. After examining my X-ray, then bending my leg backwards and sideways as I lay on the couch, he gave me the news that I had severe arthritis in my right hip and that the only answer to the problem was a titanium hip replacement. The consultant's letter to my GP includes the statement:

> ... On close examination the X-ray reveals a loss of the
> medial joint space which I think is a result of Marilyn's
> cortisol replacement therapy.

A strange time followed, a sort of limbo as I recovered from my operation, which took place only a week after my consultation. I can still see the smiling face of my surgeon looking down at me seconds before the anaesthetic took effect. As expected, I was given an injection of 100 mg of cortisol. The anaesthetist was very aware of my condition so ready to adjust the dose if necessary. Mr N told me hip replacement operations involve brutal surgery which explains the need for morphine afterwards. I remember waking up in the recovery room in a strange state of mind, calling out for my daughters and my favourite uncle. I soon discovered I was connected to a drip, tubes for morphine and blood-draining tubes which were stuck inside my right leg. What a sight! Mr N informed me I had 'a horrible hip'; the ball joint shiny through friction. Yet, despite everything, I felt so fortunate to be in such comfortable surroundings with a fascinating view from my window of London Bridge and the river Thames, an outlook that hugely contributed to my speedy recovery. I would watch from morning until dusk, a combination of busy human life as people crossed the bridge to and from their place of work, coupled with the calm flow of the river, itself busy with water vehicles of various kinds. I even attempted a sketch of St Paul's cathedral as I sat by the window of my room. I wonder what happened to that drawing?

I was made to get up and out of bed the day after my operation when an enthusiastic physiotherapist arrived to start me off on my walking programme. This began with the aid of a Zimmer frame but the next day I was handed a pair of crutches and told to use those instead! Once I could manage walking up and down stairs I was allowed to go home. I was overwhelmed by the love and support I received from everyone, which gave me such strength. Once home I developed a routine of walking around the house as well as outside; first as far as my local post box then extending it in stages until I could manage to walk comfortably around the block, using my walking stick less and less often. The strange thing was I was still in pain but now in my lower back, neck, arms and left leg but put this down to my body readjusting to its new 'limb'. I had a simple routine and enjoyed catching up on my reading. The incredible tiredness of the first six weeks lifted to see me getting out to two parties, although I declined to dance! By the time springtime came around the headteacher of my primary school telephoned to say they would be willing to adapt to suit any physical needs I may have, for example providing low chairs, and that I could go back teaching mornings only until I became used to the pace again. I was encouraged by this and planned to return in September, if not before.

It was a bit of a blow to have pain continuing in my lower back, especially after being given the all clear by my surgeon but physiotherapy helped as did a little swimming. And there was a breakthrough as by the end of March I was able to put a sock on my right foot and tie shoe laces! The pain in my lower back seemed to be lifting, just in time for my MA presentation at the Royal Festival Hall.

September arrived and I was back at school working only a few hours, gradually building up my time to three days a week. I was excited about working with children who needed support in developing their English. I remember the face of one anxious child very clearly, that of a young traumatised refugee boy from Kosovo. Initially, it was obvious from his playground behaviour that he had witnessed terrible violence during the war there but, in time, he adjusted to socialising with others, loved learning and made great strides with his English.

It wasn't long before I became restless and applied for the post of Special Needs Co-ordinator working three days a week in a very run-down London primary school which had failed its Ofsted inspection and was in Special Measures. I got the job, probably because no one else had been daft enough to apply for it! Yet for some time I had wanted to have a responsible role with children with special educational needs so, wisely or not, I left my comfortable position teaching children with English as their second language, to take on who knows what, although I knew it would involve tackling emotional and behavioural problems, as well as learning difficulties, with my new pupils. Yoga, and Pilates kept me fitter than I may have been as did regular visits to the physiotherapist as my sacrum and my neck were becoming a bit of a challenge. Life was so busy too and I had to remind myself to stand and stare so that I could ground myself and breathe! Doing regular exercises helped considerably and by the end of 2000 I was feeling more confident with myself physically.

The year 2001 seemed a lifetime away when the film *2001: A Space Odyssey* was released in 1968 and I remember thinking aloud, at the tender age of 20, 'I'll be old by then!' Well, here I was, a month away from my fifty-third birthday (not old at all) reading a review of my hip that showed everything was healing well. Life continued to be busy and fulfilling. It was of course the year of the terrorist attack on New York, the aftermath of which made everyone feel the world would never be the same again. Close to the end of the year my favourite Beatle, George Harrison, died and I wept, not only for him but for a past filled with the unique sounds and experiences the music of the fab four had brought to my generation. The wonderful thing is these sounds still live on and probably will do so for many years to come.

My diary entries gradually became more and more concise but I do note that the bone density scan result of October 2002 shows that the results are slightly below average. Although the comment reads:

> The absolute value in the left total hip has not
> changed since 1997. The absolute value of the spine
> has improved mildly since the previous scan.

I was now taking HRT in the form of Elleste Duet Conti which would be protecting my bones, for the time being at least. I was advised to stop taking HRT once I turned sixty. This I did, as I was warned that continuing to take it could result in heart problems.

School politics! 'Get me out of here' my mind kept telling me. I actually listened and escaped to the country for a few days where I spent time walking and talking with a dear friend and deciding what to do next. Despite the offer of another post in a different school, I thought it best to have a complete break. Besides, the extra stress very often meant extra hydrocortisone, which I wanted to avoid! I seemed to be holding some of this stress in my back muscles so needed to see my physiotherapist regularly. Body: 'Come on, Marilyn, it makes sense to stop!' Mind: 'But … yes, you are right!'

Family life was an exciting whirl of activity. This was the year that Esther started studying at University and Rachel began attending Sixth Form College, when Louis lost his job but fortunately soon found another, and when we adopted two cats named Alfie and Fizz who brought with them fun and entertainment as only cats can do!

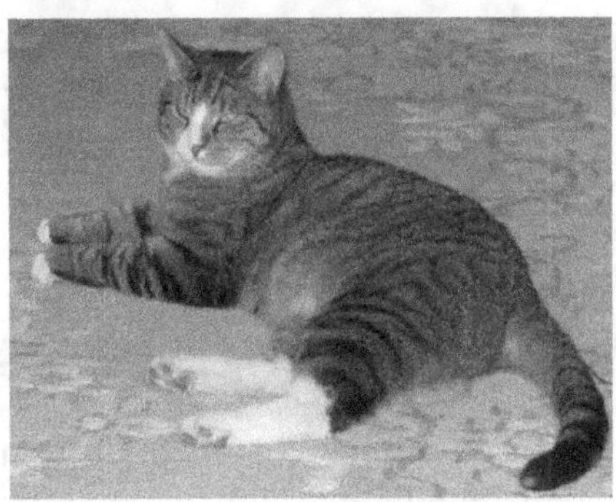

Alfie

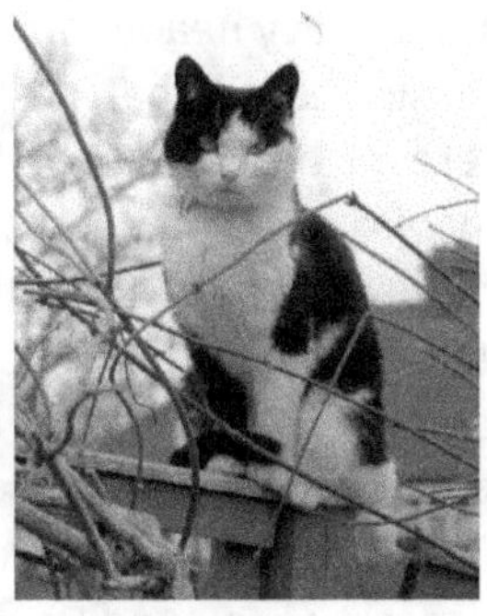

Fizz

Every week, month and year brought with it world news of change in every respect and 2003 was no exception. The uncertainty of war with Iraq loomed large in newspaper headlines as I recovered from foot surgery. The big toe on my left foot had been attacked by osteoarthritis and I had what is beautifully termed, 'a Kessel Bonny osteotomy with internal fixation', or bone surgery. Soon I would be able to move my toe up and down again and walk comfortably. As I sat with my foot propped up on a stool, snow fell heavily, creating a quiet space far removed from events beyond. The cats curled up, welcoming the warmth behind closed doors.

February arrived and with it the news I'd been half expecting yet partially dreading. Louis, who had been for some years a reservist in the Royal Navy, was mobilised and expected to board a ship bound for the Gulf. Millions of people from cities across the globe marched in peaceful protest against war but, as we know, to no avail. Since being mobilised Louis had spent time training at the Royal Naval base in Portsmouth and was now a full member of the Royal Navy. This was an emotional time for all the family as we waited for news. What actually transpired was not expected but it was quite a relief to hear that he would not be sailing anywhere but would be deployed as an ICT troubleshooter at Royal Navy headquarters in Northwood, London. Within a few days we heard that he was on 24 hours' notice to leave for wherever he was needed, possibly Kuwait, although this didn't transpire as he managed to resolve a problem they had on their computer system over the telephone. He was on shift work, barely getting any sleep and wouldn't be home for three weeks, except for weekends. In the meantime our eldest at University was suffering from repeated bouts of 'flu and tonsillitis while I was recovering from bronchitis and taking a high dose of hydrocortisone. And Dr N told me that people with my condition should try to avoid stress! I know now that it is more a case of how one handles stress. By the end of April Louis was demobilised from the Royal Navy having been offered a job in the City, and everyone's health seemed to improve. So, onwards and upwards as we put the past behind, as one must.

At the end of August Dr N examined me and thought I had experienced an adrenal low, which was perhaps not surprising, so advised me to increase my hydrocortisone for a while. Louis was travelling a great deal and I was busy visiting universities with Rachel. I also needed to fit in a hysteroscopy but thankfully there were no awful findings and it simply seemed a matter of adjusting my HRT. The following month I started teaching adults basic literacy skills. After teaching in various primary schools this was a job where I could pace myself much more easily and it only demanded two days a week of my time. Yet, by the end of the year I was off to see my physiotherapist again as my lower back was troubling me.

7

More surgery!

We must embrace pain and burn it as fuel for our journey
Kenji Miyazawa

By May 2004, and after many physiotherapy sessions, it was time to see a rheumatologist, especially as I was experiencing severe lower back pain which was becoming quite disabling. Pain was accumulating with exercise allowing me limited standing or sitting tolerances as well as difficulty in bending forward to brush my teeth! In addition, pain was radiating into both legs. The rheumatologist's report to my GP showed:

> ... a right sacroiliac joint dysfunction with associated
> lumbar spine pain and bilateral neural tension.

It was decided I needed an MRI. The result of this was reassuring except for marked degeneration change and a disc lesion at L5/S1. July arrived but further physiotherapy was not making any difference so I was referred to a consultant neurosurgeon at a spinal clinic in London. On examination the consultant advised that I was:

> markedly tender over 5/1 disc and guarded in all
> movements and has pain reproduction on flexion
> stressing of the lumbar spine. Tender anteriorly over
> 5/1 disc and also slightly at 4/5. The results of an MRI
> shows degenerative minor changes at L4/5. At L5/S1
> there is a collapsed degenerative disc which is bulging
> markedly anteriorly and bulging in the midline
> posteriorly as well. No neural compression.

A rehabilitation programme was recommended to get me fit for surgical treatment which involved going to my local swimming pool early each morning with a woggle tucked under my arm! I was to hold onto this in the water and kick my legs to strengthen the muscles as I traversed the pool, carefully avoiding serious swimmers who were no doubt irritated by my intrusion as they performed their daily lengths. Now, I was never a fan of the water, being in it or on it that is, although I had enjoyed hydrotherapy and swimming in shallow pools. Give me a winding river or vast ocean to view any day but please don't ask me to get in! But I gave it some effort and determination, hoping for an improvement in my muscle strength. Sadly, all my efforts over several weeks were in vain. Nothing changed so the woggle was relegated to the garden shed and forgotten.

Surgery loomed large on the horizon as it seemed alternatives were no longer an option. I wondered whether I could have done anything to avoid this but it all happened at such a fast pace that, despite trying various therapies, my bones were in defiance. The consultant's letter to my rheumatologist dated 17 August 2004 advises:

> In view of the extensive collapse she would probably
> be better off with a fusion rather than a disc
> replacement which I would do anteriorly in her case
> but I would want a discogram to see how badly
> affected the 3/4 and 4/5 discs are.

Meanwhile the pain was worsening. Following an MRI in October, degenerative changes at L4/5 and a gross collapse at L5/S1 with diffuse medial bulging were observed, as well as postural changes and marked tenderness on the right-sided sacroiliac joint.

Following the discogram (diagnostic radiology) to determine the anatomical source of my low back pain, my GP received this report from the consultant:

> ... the bad news is while L2/3 disc was normal the
> three discs below this all cause typical concordant
> back pain. L5/S1 disc is certainly the worst but at low

intradiscal pressure concordant pain was reproduced
at L3/4 and L4/5 as well. The best way forward would
probably be a three level disc replacement.

However, the problem was that despite success with such an operation, insurance companies would not give their support and the practice was finding great difficulty in obtaining funding for disc replacement surgery even though it was C.E. mark approved (in compliance with the applicable EU regulations) and licensed in the USA.

My insurance company confirmed that, while they would cover the cost of a spinal fusion, cover would not extend to disc replacements especially as they had not, at that time, been approved by NICE (National Institute for Health and Care Excellence).

I spent time reading vast amounts of material on the pros and cons of disc replacement but was encouraged by the number of successful operations that had taken place. I was also interested in having a second opinion. If I were to embark on such major surgery it was important that I had as much information as possible at my disposal and to feel absolutely at ease with the surgeon who was to perform this intrusive work on my body.

After my request for a second opinion, I was referred to Mr L, consultant spinal surgeon at London Bridge Hospital. A few days later when I walked into his consultation room, my intuition told me that this was the surgeon I would choose. Here was the person I could trust to cut me open, perform the repairs needed and stitch me back together again. Somehow Louis and I would find the extra cost for this procedure which, despite the risks, could give me my life back.

Mr L's diagnosis confirmed that of the previous consultant and included the observation that I had a high disability score of 76% and a low back pain score of 9/10. He added that:

> ... all activities of daily living are severely affected and
> unrelieved with both Tramadol and DF118 (an opioid
> painkiller). She has exhausted all forms of non-
> operative treatment which includes physiotherapy,
> osteopathy, acupuncture, Pilates and hydrotherapy.
> There is an element of right-sided groin pain which
> implicate L4/5 disc degeneration.

So that he could see exactly for himself what was going on, another discography was necessary which confirmed pain at L3/4 and L4/5. Mr L thought it likely that L5/S1 disc level was also causing significant low back discomfort. His letter concluded:

> I will bring her in for three level disc surgeries. This will
> entail AP fusion at L5/S1 and disc replacements at L3/4
> and L4/5.

Thoughts, fears, decisions and making the right ones kept me awake at night, as well as the pain which the drugs I was taking eased but did not remove and which at times became unbearable. Meanwhile support from my wonderful family and friends kept me going despite darker days which led me to write even darker words, gloomy yet cathartic:

> A bone screams and sets off another...
> The shrinking jelly between it and its
> neighbour allowing them to join, embrace
> and burn.
> First a mere tingle then a hotter sensation,
> growing, challenging any bonfire.
> Then, snap, the brittle bone breaks, one after
> another they go.
> Snap your fingers, snap, snap, until a pile of
> white, chalk-like pieces lies heaving,
> breathing for a while, then silence.
> My back screams but maybe not tomorrow?
> Tomorrow comes and with it teasing.
> One day an open road with a view of spaces,

the next fences barring the way
as pain shifts in its shape and form.
I cope so well and then fall into the depths of
frustration and despair...
Only to rise again!

I greeted 14 December, the day of my operation, with a drugged optimism as my head reacted to yet more opiate medication. I remember coming round feeling quite 'high' on morphine, much to Louis' surprise. Mr L gave me the news that he wasn't able to place a disc in L3/4 as the space between the discs was too small but, as he had re-aligned my spine, I shouldn't have much of a problem. I now had three screws in L5/S1 following an anterior-posterior fusion and one Prodisc in L4/5. I decided there and then to learn to love my disc (imagine a tiny version of a round, alien space ship!) and to view it as a welcome addition rather than an intruder, although seeing the X-ray affected me on all levels: mentally, emotionally and physically. After a few days I was allowed to go home, just in time to enjoy the warmth and fun of a family Christmas.

A new pain introduced itself on Christmas day which I reported to my surgeon on my follow-up visit a few days later. This was symmetrical, running down both legs and burned like nerves on fire. Mr L gave me some medication to ease this pain although I can't remember what it was.

By the time 2005 arrived I record having short local walks as I remained quite stiff yet uplifted by everyone's thoughts and love which helped me so much when I felt I was not getting better quickly enough! The pain I was experiencing was moving around and was particularly strong in my leg muscles and nerves. By February it began to change in nature and intensity as well as location. It would be three months before I would be able to return to work but I was in no rush. My surgeon was pleased with my progress but thought an injection of cortisone into a specific facet joint in my spine (facet joints are located in the back and neck at each vertebral level) would provide relief from the pain and inflammation I was experiencing in the lower part of my back. Sitting was proving difficult as I needed to get up and move around almost every half an hour then try a different chair. I was assured by Mr L that the pain emanating from the facet joints was not serious and that I would continue to improve once the L5/S1 fusion started to take. The facet joint injection actually increased the level of pain but by June, and after sessions of Pilates and physiotherapy, I found I had a new lease of life with few aches and pains and was experiencing only some mild left trochanteric bursitis. My X-rays showed L5/S1 interbody fusion and no subsidence of the L4/5 disc replacement. I felt I was at last getting my life back despite my neck and shoulders complaining and reacting to my new posture!

August, and time for another bone density scan. This time the results showed osteopenia, slight thinning of the bones.

One wonders why, when I was recovering so well, feeling strong and full of optimism, that a man, tripping on a step while entering a coffee shop where I was enjoying ordering a cappuccino, crashes into my back, bounces off me and onto the floor. Leaving my unpaid for goods at the counter, I found a chair outside and sat down to recover from the shock and quickly took an extra dose of hydrocortisone. I won't go into details of what, or rather what was not, recorded by the staff or the legalities than ensued which came to nothing, but four days later my left leg went from under me as I was about to step into a busy road. As with the accident, I immediately increased my hydrocortisone dose again to deal with the shock and continued on this higher dose for a few days until I felt comfortable. Just to make sure all was well, I returned earlier than previously arranged to see Mr L and also saw my osteopath. Mr L assured me that no obvious dislocation of the disc replacement had occurred following the accident and that the fusion was also sound but this awful event meant that I needed to wear a sacroiliac belt for a while for support. My main problem, he noted, was sitting intolerance but I decided I would rather soldier on with this than have facet joint injections.

It's amazing what one can do and my diary is full of events including my decision to move on from teaching in the adult education sector and to take a post working with a Hospital School and Outreach Centre. In December Mr L reported my delight with the outcome of my surgery and that I now had minimal back pain. With great relief I was able to agree that I had returned to living a completely normal life and was very able-bodied! My preoperative ODI (Oswestry Disability Index) score had been 76%, i.e. severe disability. Now it was 12%, i.e. mild disability. My preoperative back pain score had been 9/10 but was now 1.5/10. My X-rays were satisfactory. I imagined myself being like a phoenix rising from the ashes and beginning to soar, with occasional desperate flapping of wings to keep me going, a nervous drop and then up again, to where the air is sweeter.

8

A holistic approach

A cure of the parts should not be attempted without treatment of the whole

Plato

Physical parts of me were certainly being treated and had been for some time, not only my pituitary condition but those parts operated on, each one separately by different specialists bringing their knowledge and skills to perform amazing work, putting my body back together again. But for as long as I can remember I have known that there is more to us than the physical body. We are made up of energy which flows through everything but it is also possible to tap into that energy which is healing and restorative. For many years I had been conscious of my own and other people's energy fields as well as a healing white light flooding through me when meditating. I now wanted to discover more with the initial aim of supporting and complementing my physical healing. I found this in the form of Reiki, life energy that moves through the body during treatments. As it flows it removes blocked energy due to stress or illness, allowing the body to relax completely so that healing can take place.

My discovery came about through a number of meaningful coincidences, or synchronicities, when seemingly random experiences put me on the right path. Very quickly, from thinking about developing in this direction, I unexpectedly met a lady who spoke to me about Reiki and its benefits. My curiosity led me to doing some research using the internet, as well as reading various books. There were many Reiki schools advertising on the internet but time and time again I kept returning to one particular school: Reiki Evolution. The more I read, the more I felt comfortable with their approach.

In March 2006 I completed my First Degree Reiki course with one of Reiki Evolution's Reiki Masters, spending a few days studying prior to the practical training day. On the day, I was given an Empowerment, along with the other students present. Reiki Empowerments, or Attunements, give us permission to recognise what is already within but which we have forgotten exists. Once we receive an empowerment or attunement we are able to channel Reiki energy, not just for our own benefit but for the benefit of others. I found the daily meditations and self-healing exercises energising and friends remarked on how relaxed and calm they felt after I had given them a hands-on treatment. When I fell and injured my leg my osteopath came to the rescue. To my delight she told me she also practised Reiki which explained why her hands always felt so hot! Whenever physical problems reminded me of their presence, practising Reiki and giving myself treatments, allowed me to step back and welcome the calmness it brought in order to deal with them.

The founder of Reiki, Mikao Usui, grew up in a Tendai Buddhist family in Japan between 1865 and 1926. He referred to it as a 'method to achieve personal perfection'. His approach is simple and I'd like to pass on to you his Reiki Precepts which, when practised regularly, allow one to let go, to a huge degree, the stresses of life that cause physical, mental, spiritual and emotional pain and discomfort.

> The secret art of inviting happiness. The miraculous
> medicine of all diseases:
> Just for today (which exhorts us to be fully engaged
> in the moment, to be mindful)
> Do not anger,
> Do not worry
> Be humble
> Be honest (in your dealings with other people)
> Be compassionate towards yourself and others.

As I wanted very much to develop my Reiki practice, three months after completing my Reiki 1 course I embarked on my second degree course, which meant it was possible for me to channel energies focusing on the physical and emotional needs of the recipient (including myself).

I continued to practise Reiki not only on myself but on family and friends and we all experienced the benefits this energy gave us as it helped our bodies and minds to heal. In her book entitled *The NHS Healer* Angie Buxton-King[8] talks about how orthodox medicine and complementary alternative therapies work together. She succeeded in persuading University College hospital in London to allow her to treat some of their patients, resulting in the hospital continuing to offer cancer patients Reiki, together with other therapies, to help with their recovery or in assisting near the end of their lives. It is interesting to learn that Scientists are now beginning to show an interest in energy medicine such as Reiki, magnet therapy and acupuncture, as illustrated in *Energy Medicine* by James L. Oschman[9]:

> Oschman … noted the similarity between the
> frequencies and intensities of low energy emissions
> from the hands of therapists and the signals from
> pulsed electromagnetic field devices used in clinical
> medicine.

In September I began teaching at the local Hospital School and Outreach Service working with young teenagers who were either school refusers or who suffered from severe medical conditions. By the end of the year Mr L discharged me but referred me to a physiotherapist as my neck was giving me trouble. It appeared that my upper back was taking extra strain after what had been done below. His letter to my GP states:

> Marilyn is just short of two years following her L4/5
> disc replacement and L5/S1 posterior fusion. She had
> done brilliantly and is leading a normal life. She gets
> the occasional twinge and recently had a mild spell of
> left-sided back pain which settled after a period of

> intense walking while on holiday in Prague!
>
> X-rays are very satisfactory showing no evidence of
> metal work failure and she has a beautifully aligned
> spine. She does have occasional muscle tension in her
> neck so I have referred her to physiotherapy.

Physiotherapy was beneficial but I was also getting better at mindfully channelling Reiki energy towards my pain or discomfort, enabling it to ease to quite an extent. It also made a significant difference in helping me come to terms with what was going on.

Early the following year, I re-visited Mr L who ordered an MRI of my neck. This scan showed multi-level disc degeneration affecting C3/4 down to C7/T1. I was offered cervical trigger point and facet injections but declined. In time my body seemed to adjust to the problem and the pain eased. Today it still troubles me but I have a fair range of movement and can still turn my head when reversing my car! I have to thank my osteopath and Alexander Technique practitioner (like my osteopath, another Reiki healer) for their contributions.

It is reassuring to know there are complementary therapies out there which can help us deal with problems encountered when the body goes wrong! A holistic approach considers the 'whole' person, treating not just the symptoms and the problem. This approach looks at a person's physical, mental, emotional and spiritual needs to achieve optimal health and wellness. Reiki, osteopathy, yoga and acupuncture are a few of these therapies. My GP recognises the benefits of Reiki and an acupuncturist is available at the surgery. I'm sure that the more orthodox and complementary therapies work together, the greater the benefit will be for all.

Another energy technique I came across, introduced to me by a Reiki colleague, was EFT (Emotional Freedom Techniques) or what many people may recognise as the Tapping procedure. This technique allows the recipient to find the emotional source behind their pain by tapping on various acupressure points of the head and shoulders. It looks quite bizarre yet has amazing results as it works on shifting the problem. Having been impressed with what I saw and experienced personally, I decided to train to be a practitioner. Shortly after making this decision, I decided I was ready to study for the Reiki Master Teacher level and qualified in April 2007. A new road lay ahead as I planned my new 'career'. My work with the hospital school was intermittent so I decided to rent a therapy room to practise Reiki and EFT, and in September 2007 I found one that was fairly local. I would practice there two mornings a week. At first business was slow but after setting up a website and focusing on some marketing, people started to trickle in through the doors. I loved this work and once I retired from teaching in February 2008 I was able to work longer hours and begin teaching Reiki, soon moving to therapy rooms in Victoria, central London where clients came along for Reiki, EFT or Reiki training. Reiki students came to me through my own website but a great opportunity presented itself when I was asked by the director of Reiki Evolution (who was looking for a Reiki teacher to practise in central London) if I would be happy to join his team of teachers. I gladly accepted and continued to be part of this wonderful team for five years.

9

More surprises!

The greatest glory in living lies not in never falling, but rising every time we fall
Nelson Mandela

It was certainly a time of change both at work and at home, now very quiet as our daughters were travelling together for a few months to strange and exotic places. We looked forward with great anticipation to their regular emails up until their safe return in April 2008, two months after my sixtieth birthday. Feeling inspired by the girls, Louis and I began to plan a trip to Australia and New Zealand for later in the year, travelling via Hong Kong and returning via California where we would stay with friends. But these plans were immediately put on hold for a year when we learned in August that my dear brother had been diagnosed with a cancerous tumour on the base of his tongue. I wasn't going anywhere while he had to endure chemotherapy and radiotherapy for this type 3 cancer. John accepted the situation with great stoicism while the family were devastated, yet hopeful. I'm sure many families in such situations feel quite helpless and so did we, but we needed to be strong for him. All we could do was support him, pray and I could ask for Reiki healing to help him get through his ordeal. By December and after his gruelling treatment, his throat was still too swollen for an examination so he had to wait until February 2009 to hear that he was 99.5% clear, although he needed an operation to open the back of his throat so he could eat. He has survived, but to this day he carries the physical and emotional scars of the lifesaving but severe treatment he received.

During this period of time any difficulties I may have had paled into insignificance. All I have to report is the result of another bone density scan showing that it was better than before but not normal. There was still evidence of osteopenia.

Despite the economic crisis of 2008 I managed to keep my little business afloat and in November 2009 Louis and I took ourselves off on the trip we had planned the previous year.

January 2010 arrived and at last we seemed to be coming out of the Big Freeze that had dominated our weather that winter. Our trip had been more than uplifting and had given me the impetus to go on with my Reiki practice for an indefinite period of time. The energy generated with each Reiki course and treatment continued to flow and I felt I was in a very different place to where I had been a few years earlier, so much so that I embarked on a training course in cognitive hypnotherapy with the Quest Institute which had been recommended by Reiki colleagues. My mind was ready to learn something new and add another helpful therapy to my list. By 2011, having completed some months of study and attending weekend courses, I qualified as a cognitive hypnotherapist, and incorporated this therapy into my practice.

By now, Dr N had retired and I was under the care of another endocrinologist, Dr P at Guy's hospital. At our first session he arranged a full pituitary hormone profile, commenting in his letter to my GP that I was on a relatively generous dose of hydrocortisone by today's standards and depending on my results would consider reducing this a little. He thought I appeared well but with slightly thin skin. Otherwise there were no overt signs of over replacement of glucocorticoids and my pituitary hormone profile suggested adequate replacement therapy. Dr P suggested I take 125 mcg of thyroxine daily rather than alternating the dose as I had been doing. He reminded me about the need to increase my hydrocortisone therapy at times of illness and to seek medical help if I experienced vomiting and was unable to tolerate my hydrocortisone tablets.

In September yet another bone density scan showed that,

according to the World Health Organization guidelines, I had low bone mass and was considered to be osteopenic. Again I wondered whether my medical condition had anything to do with this. I also questioned how much ageing came into the equation, having read that after the menopause (although I didn't have one) women can lose 30% of their bone mass.

The highlight of the following year was, for many, the 2012 Olympics in London. How exhilarating this was for both those involved in the events and crowds alike and no one will forget its spectacular opening ceremony. This was a much needed boost, bringing people of all nations and parts of the country together to share the excitement. My policeman nephew spent the happiest two or three weeks of his career on duty there – no arrests were necessary! The atmosphere in London was palpable.

Around this time I had been reading about growth hormone and was just a bit perturbed to read that someone with my condition should have it prescribed to them. I think everyone is aware that this hormone controls growth in children but many people I have spoken to are unaware that it is also involved in the maintenance of normal body weight, muscle and bone strength, and well-being in adults. I was particularly interested to note the inclusion of its role in muscle and bone strength as I could relate this to the lowering of my bone density scores as well as weakness I had felt for some time in my leg and arm muscles. Some years previously I had been asked certain questions by Dr N which I seem to remember related to my quality of life but, on examining the results, he didn't seem to think I had a problem. At that time I was still taking HRT so maybe this affected the results, as taking it would have made me feel less tired. Now, however, despite feeling I was in a good place and able to deal well with life, I was beginning to be aware of an underlying lack of energy. I decided to ask Dr P on my next visit whether I should be taking growth hormone. When I did so, he ordered a blood test which was followed by an insulin tolerance test. This test is used to produce extreme hypoglycaemia to assess the amount of growth hormone released as part of the stress mechanism.

This isn't something I would want to repeat! It wasn't so much having insulin injected into a vein in my hand and having my blood glucose measured at regular intervals that bothered me. As I became more and more hypoglycaemic I gradually began to feel I was saying goodbye to the world, just managing to call out, 'Bring me back to normal!' to the team of excellent nurses. Miraculously, at the end of the test, one glass of a fizzy glucose drink did the trick and I came back to life almost immediately! After drinking one more glass of this wonderful elixir, and eating a somewhat battered sandwich which I'd carried to the hospital with me, I had my blood pressure checked, sat for a while to rest, then was allowed to return home.

While waiting for the results of the insulin tolerance test, I found new, very quirky but adequate therapy rooms close to Victoria station where I continued to enjoy working with a variety of clients. I was quite busy and enjoying the buzz generated by it all but, nevertheless, it was time for a break so, in October 2012 Louis and I took ourselves off to the beautiful, rugged county of Northumberland, bordering the county of Durham where I spent the first fourteen years of my life. We had found ourselves a castle – well, not exactly, we were renting the gatehouse of a castle in Morpeth. The renovation of this ancient building had retained the building's features and stone coldness but, thank goodness, central heating had been tastefully installed. I was aware of much energy in the rooms and my hands would tingle, more in some rooms than others! Despite it only being October, I remember viewing from our cosy room early morning frosts glistening on the grass outside under golden red sunrises. We were joined soon after our arrival by our youngest daughter and her boyfriend, their presence injecting much fun and conversation. So, after a few days of breathing the bracing, fresh air and only just avoiding being blown into the sea, it was time to return, collect our cat from the cattery (sadly, only Alfie now) and resume our busy lives.

On our return to the city, I found my GP had received the result of my insulin tolerance test.

> As expected, the insulin test shows she (Marilyn) is completely growth hormone deficient … growth hormone levels throughout the test remained completely undetectable at <0.1 µg/L … there is no doubt she fulfils the NICE criteria for severe growth hormone deficiency and therefore warrants a trial of growth hormone therapy.

Because my quality of life was seen to be impaired by growth hormone deficiency, I also needed to complete a Quality of Life Assessment of Growth Hormone Deficiency in Adults and this was done at regular intervals with my endocrine nurse to measure improvements in my scores. I was given twenty-five statements such as 'I have to struggle to finish jobs' and 'I avoid mixing with people I don't know well' and had to answer 'yes' or 'no' to these. My endocrinologist prescribed Somatropin, 5 mg/1.5 ml cartridges with a starting dose of 0.2 mg using the NordiPen device, to be injected into my abdomen each evening. By December I was injecting 0.3 mg of growth hormone daily and noticing a definite improvement in my well-being as well as an increase in my energy levels. While all this was going on I had the (hopefully never to be repeated) adrenal crisis which I describe in Chapter 3!

I don't seem to have recorded much in 2013 except for nagging myself to write more (even if it was only diary notes), and visiting Guy's hospital regularly where I was being monitored by Dr P, my endocrinologist, and my endocrine nurse. In February, after three months on growth hormone I was asked to increase my dose to 0.4 mg once daily and this is the dose I continue to inject each evening. After a thyroid function test, Dr P reduced my thyroxine dose from 125 mcg to 100 mcg. I felt better on this lower dose as at times I had felt as though I was 'racing'! It was also hoped that growth hormone therapy would improve my bone density. In August my endocrine nurse wrote to my GP to let him know that my IGF-1 (marker for growth hormone) was in the upper half of the normal range. My QoL AGHDA score had decreased from 14/25 to 3/25 reflecting a positive change in my quality of life. She also noted that I met the NICE criteria for continuation of growth hormone therapy (NICE criteria recommends an improvement of AGHDA score of 7).

It was a relief to be taking growth hormone at last and to be receiving the correct dose. While my endocrinologist assured me that this hormone helps bone density and muscles to improve, he has recently confirmed that lack of growth hormone in the past may have increased the risk of thinning of my bones. I am also aware that other symptoms of lack of growth hormone include impaired concentration and memory and a decrease in the amount of muscle bulk and strength.

Towards the end of the year Louis and I took ourselves off to Dubrovnik in Croatia, somewhere we had often thought about visiting. We spent two weeks there, travelling to Bosnia and Montenegro and resorts along the sparkling Adriatic coastline. This must be the most beautiful coastline I have ever seen, the extraordinary light exposing various shades of green and blue on land and sea. Dubrovnik is very hilly and should perhaps carry a health warning for those with dodgy backs! Half way through our holiday I was struggling to climb the hill up to our rented apartment and needed to rely more and more on taxi rides home.

Shortly after returning home from holiday, I began to feel bothered by the nagging pain in my lower back which, despite gentle exercises and Pilates, wasn't going away. It seemed that the best course of action was to see Mr L, the spinal surgeon who had performed my disc replacement and fusion in 2004. His letter dated November 2013 to my GP gives the unexpected news that:

> … there is a pseudarthrosis (the result of a failed spinal
> fusion) at L5/S1. Marilyn was a little bit shocked by
> this but I have explained that <1% of fusions go on to a
> non-union. This is more common typically at the L5/S1
> segment.

This certainly did take me by surprise! The proposed treatment was that I needed:

> Removal metalwork and revision L5/S1 instrumented
> posterolateral fusion/ anterior posterior fusion (risks
> of surgery include <1% of infection, bleeding, nerve
> root injury, cauda equine syndrome, fusion failure,
> metalwork failure, revision surgery, DVT, PE and
> pneumonia).

I thought it best to put the risks out of my head!

I was admitted to London Bridge Hospital on the 12 December 2013. Again, I had an injection of 100 mg of cortisol before my operation. After yet another December operation, by the 15th my physiotherapist and surgeon agreed that I could go home, which was a relief as Christmas was on the horizon and I obviously wanted to spend it in the comfort of my own home with my family. I left hospital wondering what happened to make those screws in my lower back, once so well fused, decide to detach themselves. Surely, it couldn't simply have been due to walking up those steep hills in Dubrovnik! Mr L had replaced the screws with a new solution, which was expected to hold. I crossed my fingers in the hope that it would! So, another hill to climb but maybe a minor one when compared with what many have to endure. I was reminded of another quotation by Nelson Mandela, who passed away just before I had my operation:

> After climbing a great hill, one only finds that there are
> many more hills to climb.

I saw Mr L again six weeks after my operation and was more than pleased to hear that my wounds had healed up nicely and I was making slow and steady progress. I had been experiencing short, sharp shooting pains on my left side but overall I believed that this was improving.

In March 2014 I returned for X-rays, which looked very satisfactory. Unfortunately, I had developed bilateral trochanteric bursitis which was worse on the left side, as well as some neural L5 left-sided irritation. Mr L decided it would be beneficial for me to have a steroid injection in the nerve and this seemed to do the trick. In May he informed my GP that my left L5 sciatic nerve was playing up and that I was noticing pain in my left groin which was travelling to my knee and occasionally below my knee. Mr L thought that an arthritic painful left hip was causing the symptoms as opposed to true sciatica. He also remarked that:

> ... from a lumbar point of view Marilyn's back pain has
> completely resolved with the instrumented
> posterolateral fusion with BMP [which, I learned, is
> Bone Morphogenetic Protein which stimulates the
> growth of new bone].

After a CT scan there was no evidence of problems with the fusion or that there may be narrowing of the disc space or bone spurs. Mr L advised that I should have a left hip injection (diagnostic and hopefully therapeutic). If it resolved my left leg pain then he would surmise that this was secondary to left hip osteoarthritis. He also ordered a nerve conduction study on my pending hip injection.

Surprising results followed, or maybe they weren't! Here is what Mr L wrote to my GP in July:

> It is quite clear Marilyn's hip is causing the problem.
> She has lost joint space on her pelvic X-ray. The hip
> injection offered a few days of relief but now the pains
> have returned with a vengeance.

He referred me to a colleague, Mr G, who was to be my hip surgeon.

I was greeted warmly by this friendly surgeon who immediately put me at ease. Shortly after my consultation in June, Mr G wrote a lengthy letter to my GP outlining the pain I was experiencing and the treatment I'd had so far. He remarked that I walked with a mild antalgic gait, which I understood meant a gait that develops to avoid pain when walking, and that I was Trendelenburg positive. What a wonderful term. What it meant was that when standing on one leg, my pelvis dropped on the side opposite to that leg, indicating muscle weakness. It was decided that a total hip replacement was on the cards but there were certain events that I had to think about, the most important being our eldest daughter's wedding which was to be in early August. I couldn't miss that. I'd even bought my hat! The next issue was that Louis and I had already booked a special holiday to visit friends in Hawaii in November and Mr G explained that, to avoid blood clots, I must wait three months after the operation before undertaking a major long-haul flight. I have to say again how fortunate I was to have the choice of an operation date, all down to me being eligible to use Louis' company's health cover. I know of people who don't have this privilege and who have had to wait months in agonising pain before having their hip replacement operation. My operation was booked for 18 August, ten days after our daughter's wedding which turned out to be a wonderful day when the sun shone brightly and everyone celebrated.

Mr G communicated with my endocrinologist who advised that I should stop injecting growth hormone on the day of surgery and only restart it when I left hospital. He emphasised that I would need hydrocortisone cover, having intravenous injections of 50 mg six hourly, starting with the induction of anaesthetic. Once I was eating and drinking relatively normally I could be transferred back to oral hydrocortisone which should initially be around 20 mg four times a day, reducing gradually to my normal dose as I recovered. Ten days after my operation Mr G informed my GP that my hip replacement was uneventful. I remember him appearing shortly after my operation and thanking me for being a 'text book case.' It was a relief to learn, six weeks after surgery that my wound had healed well. I had experienced some bouts of back pain since my operation and sciatica down the back of my left leg but on examination there were no tension signs and the hip moved freely and painlessly. Mr G noted in a letter to my GP that the envelope around the hip was understandably a little weak, causing some aching. I was interested to find out that anyone with a mechanical back pain is likely to notice a worsening in their level of pain following a hip replacement before it begins to get better. Physiotherapy would help here and I found a highly recommended therapist who helped me enormously.

In December I found myself back at London Bridge Hospital but this time for a routine check with Mr L who had performed the delicate operation on my lower back a year previously. He happily discharged me as my X-rays looked very satisfactory. All that remained was some background aching, stiffness and minor nerve irritation.

The year 2014 had been bit of an emotional rollercoaster as we experienced the joys of a family wedding, an amazing holiday in Hawaii and the birth of my niece's first baby. This was countered by Louis being made redundant early in the year and having to think about setting up his own business, my father's death in January followed by the passing of a special uncle four months later. The wedding lifted our spirits then only a few days afterwards my brother had a triple heart by-pass operation. A week after that I had my hip surgery. Ending the year with our trip to warmer climes was uplifting to say the least.

Throughout the year I paid regular visits to my endocrinologist who sent me off for another bone density scan. The findings showed that there had been further loss of density compared to the previous study, showing a degree of osteopenia.

Somewhat reluctantly I decided I needed to have a break from my work so, close to the end of the year, I took my final Reiki workshop and saw my last clients for treatments and cognitive hypnotherapy. It was time to pause, reflect and repair.

10

Making the right choices

*To keep the body in good health is a duty … otherwise we shall not be able to keep our
mind strong and clear*

Buddha

The next two years seemed to disappear so quickly. It is a cliché to say 'time flies' yet we all seem to say it because we're under the illusion that it does! My time was taken up with a different focus, much of it enjoying time with friends and visiting the many places that London has to offer, as well as taking a few short breaks away from home. I was enjoying this new phase in my life although experiencing a little impatience as it seemed to be taking a while for my body to spring back to life.

In January 2015 I saw my hip surgeon, Mr G, who noted that I had no major problems in terms of my recovery and my X-rays were satisfactory. I was getting some discomfort in the trochanteric region (the large bump on the outside of the upper end of the femur) on both sides and some lower back and buttock pain but no true sciatica. I learned from his letter to my GP that:

> Whilst I used a posterior approach to not violate the
> abductors at all, the combination of her previous
> lumbar spinal disease and her steroids means that she
> has a couple of factors causing her abductors to
> overload.

To help remedy this problem I visited my physiotherapist, promising to practise the exercises she gave me at home.

It was a relief to learn from my hip surgeon that whereas an X-ray of my right hip, which had been replaced in 1999, showed a few early signs of wear there was certainly no imminent need for any action on this side, despite it being well past its sell-by date!

I didn't see Mr G again until August when X-rays showed a fully ingrown implant. I had been experiencing some sacroiliac pain, which my osteopath had treated, and he noted that the aching was probably a function of my previous spinal fusion. He recommended that I have an annual X-ray on my right hip to monitor any wear and tear.

In the meantime I saw my endocrinologist, Dr P, for regular reviews. In April my QoL AGHDA score was 0/25 indicating an excellent response to growth hormone replacement and no changes were necessary as far as my current endocrine replacement was concerned. I was advised that I should have another bone density scan in 2016 with a view to deciding whether or not any further intervention would be required for the osteopenia. He also arranged a hydrocortisone day curve assessment to see whether there was any scope for trying to reduce my daily dose.

This was done in June. I arrived at St Thomas' hospital feeling quite wobbly as this was a fasting blood test so I wasn't allowed to eat after 10pm the night before the test. Neither was I allowed to have any medication that morning. The day was spent lying on a bed with a cannula in my arm and blood was taken every hour from 10am until 5pm. After the first sample was taken I was asked to take my normal morning dose of hydrocortisone. It was a long day but I think I managed to get some reading done to pass the time! On my next visit to see my endocrinologist he told me the results showed that my cortisol levels rose to a relatively high level after taking my morning dose of hydrocortisone but that they dropped to quite low values at around eight hours. In light of this it was recommended that I remain on the same dose of hydrocortisone but perhaps experiment with taking my second dose a little earlier than I had been doing, which was around 6.30pm. I tried this and found that taking it at 5pm instead made a little difference to how I felt and probably helped me sleep better. However, only recently I have split my dose (as mentioned in Chapter 3) to match my circadian rhythm and now feel even better.

The year ended with the arrival of heavy rain and flooding brought by storms which battered most of the United Kingdom, with devastating results. Everyone will remember the previous month's terrorist attacks carried out at a concert hall in Paris by gunmen and suicide bombers, bringing fear and threats to us all and the world as we knew it and with more to follow.

Two thousand and sixteen arrived, a year not only to be remembered for the passing from this world of many brilliant people, but also one which would bring the unexpected results of the referendum to leave the European Union; then, a few months later, a storm of a different kind with the shock election result in the USA. In our microcosmic world it was comforting to continue living our ordinary lives, attempting to stay sane as we carried out our routine tasks, following plans and considering how fortunate we were. The greatest event for us was the birth of our first granddaughter who continues to bring joy as we watch her develop under the wise guidance of her parents.

So, back to my story and the other things that came along. In July it was time for a routine check on my 'old' hip just to make sure that there was no wear and tear going on. The X-ray showed a little of this but nothing serious. While I was there I told my surgeon about my concern that a hollow had appeared in the muscle of my left buttock. I had noticed it appearing some months after my spinal re-fusion in 2013 and really should have had the problem investigated then. What followed was communication between my two surgeons as they deliberated over whether the cause was detachment of the tendon following my hip surgery in August 2014 or whether nerve damage had occurred in the lower back following my spinal re-fusion in 2013.

(I had been warned that this surgery could trigger nerve damage). It was arranged that I should have an MRI scan of my lumbar spine and a nerve conduction study.

The nerve conduction test was not at all comfortable! Small pads were placed on my skin to record the activity of the nerves, and little electric shocks were given to the nerves elsewhere to activate them. This test did not show any detachment of the tendon but it did show chronic L5 denervation which, Mr L explained, was in keeping with my gluteal wasting. The MRI showed a very flared L4/5 segment due to the disc replacement but no overt nerve root compression. It was recommended that I needed intensive physiotherapy, i.e. gluteal strengthening exercises to assist with this wasting. My neck was also scanned and Mr L noted that this showed:

> T1–2 degenerative spondylolisthesis with foraminal
> narrowing and this would certainly explain the wasting
> in the hand intrinsics.

I had noticed this wasting between each thumb and forefinger for some time. At least it isn't painful! I continue to experience aches and stiffness in my neck but with careful exercise, including Alexander Technique, I'm not doing too badly.

Around the same time I had yet another bone density scan, the result of which showed that my T-scores had deteriorated somewhat since the last scan. I now had a T-score of –2.5 in my lumbar spine and –2.9 in my forearm. My endocrinologist explained that these were now in the osteoporotic range and advised me to start taking a weekly dose (70 mg) of the bisphosphonate alendronic acid to protect my bones. It was suggested that I would have a repeat bone density test in around 18 months' time. Otherwise a blood test showed that my free thyroid hormones were normal.

While my GP was happy to prescribe alendronic acid following

Dr P's advice, something made me think that I should do a bit of research on the efficacy and side effects of taking this drug. What were the alternatives? I talked to a lot of professional people, including my dentist, who urged me to start taking it. On hearing this advice, I felt a little reassured but remained wary as two of the rare side effects listed in the package leaflet describe unusual fracture of the thigh bone and possible pain in the jaw which could be signs of bone damage (osteonecrosis) generally associated with delayed healing and infection and usually following tooth extraction. I was advised that if I ever needed to have a tooth removed this would be carried out in hospital rather than at a dental surgery and that I would be given antibiotics to deal with any possible infection. I wasn't comfortable with this idea and decided to do more research. I spoke to three ladies who had taken this drug for up to ten years. None had experienced any side effects but two told me it hadn't made any difference to their bone density scores. In her book *Better Bones, Better Body*, Susan E Brown,[10] states that Fosamax (alendronic acid) is reported to have failed at halting bone breakdown in some 20 percent of all cases. She stresses the importance of obtaining bone density scans of the spine and hip to measure success although 'the bone density measurement cannot distinguish between bone loss that occurred in the past but has now stabilised and bone loss that is actively occurring at the time'. I spent a bit of time deliberating so that I made the right choice but finally decided to start the treatment in September, 2016. I chose a Wednesday morning for my weekly intake, swallowed my tablet as soon as I woke up and waited for half an hour, sitting upright as instructed, before eating breakfast. All seemed fine. I thought I could get used to this seemingly odd regime.

This fairly comfortable feeling of acceptance didn't last as, during week three, I noticed I was beginning to experience some pain in my upper jaw. At the time I put this down to inflammation of the temple mandibular joints which my GP had diagnosed some months earlier, which caused minor discomfort. By week four I was aware of the pain creeping down into my lower jaw, making it feel a little heavy. This worried me as I had never experienced pain here. It was all a little scary so I chose to stop taking the medication. To my relief, within a week or so, all jaw pain had disappeared and it seemed a good time to have a chat with my GP. He understood exactly how I felt but advised strongly that I must replace the alendronic acid with a serious fitness programme, including weight-bearing exercises and to include adequate nutrients in my diet (focusing on an alkaline forming diet) as well as supplements for optimal bone health. I realised it was also important to minimise any physical and emotional stress where possible and this is where meditation, relaxation and Reiki came in to support my health and bring a greater sense of calm when life became challenging! I was keen to take this alternative path and to seriously think about what was right for my body.

We are frequently told by the media, as well as professionals, that bones grow stronger if we exercise and build muscle, whereas if we are inactive bones will tend to get lighter and thinner, an alternative I wish to avoid at all costs. There have been times when I have been more inactive than I would have liked, such as when I needed to recover from an operation, but otherwise I have always been quite mobile, although not in such a concentrated fashion as I am having to be now. Some of my muscle weakness may very well be due to a lack of growth hormone in previous years. Having taken it for almost five years now, I am very hopeful that it is having a positive impact!

Calcium is of course very important to bone health and, until a few months ago, I had been taking a prescribed amount of calcium with added Vitamin D3. Information gleaned from both Susan Brown's book, and from a reputable local nutritionist, assured me that while calcium is essential for bone health, it does not stand alone. Brown explains that, 'using high doses of calcium in the face of magnesium deficiency can contribute to a depositing of calcium in the joints promoting arthritis ...'.[11] She lists as many as seventeen other nutrients that are also essential for bone health and explains that, if our diets are low in any of these, our bones suffer. I am now taking, as prescribed by my nutritionist, a bone support tablet which includes nutrients that allow for full absorption of calcium, i.e. magnesium, isoflavones, vitamin K2 (MK-7) and vitamin D3. It also made sense to check what I was eating to make sure I was consuming a balanced diet, one which was more alkaline than acidic. So I was on a mission to be more conscious than ever about the foods that I ate, as well as those to avoid, and to programme myself to be even more active. To this end I joined an hourly Walk-Fit programme in my local park where a group of us follow a trained fitness instructor, first walking slowly, then briskly, incorporating various exercises. We also manage to enjoy a good chat! I will continue with this for as long as I can keep going, together with Pilates and daily walks. Maybe I should get a dog! With time, my muscles, as well as my bones, should grow stronger or at least not become weaker. 'A useful finding,' says Susan Brown, (and which supports my earlier reference to bone health) 'is the correlation between muscle mass and bone mass. If we build muscle, we build bone. Conversely, if we lose muscle, we lose bone.'[12] Friends and I agree that the interesting thing about getting older seems to be that one needs to be conscious of doing even more to keep the body fit. The old adage 'use it or lose it' is a truism. Next year I will reach the age of seventy (how did that happen so quickly?) so I have my work cut out for me and will need to consider what the right choices are as I go! It will be interesting to see the result of the next bone density scan.

11

Summing up

The past cannot be changed. The future is yet in your power
Unknown

Many years have passed since I woke up on that November morning in 1972 with the headache to end all headaches and which heralded the beginning of my journey with hypopituitarism. I will never know for certain whether the other things that happened to come along were a result of this condition, although there does appear to be a strong connection. Writing this book has clarified a lot of things for me and has given me greater insight into how our amazing bodies function, what can go wrong with them and how, with help, they can heal.

Living with a pituitary condition can be quite challenging psychologically as well as emotionally, mentally and physically, particularly for those who suffer from a pituitary tumour and have to undergo surgery. On initial diagnosis we have to come to terms with a changed image of who we are and how this new version of ourselves will impact on our relationships, self-confidence, health, employment and well-being. Adjustments need to be made to our lifestyle and how we manage our dependency on hormone replacement. I remember Dr N telling me that because pituitary patients know that they live with a life-threatening illness, which is dependent on a strict regime of taking their tablets and what might happen if they don't, they will always suffer from some level of anxiety although they may not be conscious of this.

I realise that some pituitary conditions are far more severe, and have a larger impact on day-to-day living, than my own condition and I am thankful that, to a large degree, I can lead a normal life. But having hypopituitarism does mean that I don't always have the physical resources to do all the things I would like to do and it takes me a while to recover from illnesses or stressful situations. I enjoy socialising but find late nights exhaust me and it can be embarrassing to try to explain to people that I have to leave an event long before they themselves are ready to, particularly when I don't look tired or unwell! Although I find it difficult to tell myself to slow down, I do need to pace myself carefully and use strategies such as energy work, meditation and the practice of mindfulness to bring a sense of calm and acceptance, to boost my energy and help me remain positive at times when life seems a bit too much! I would recommend these practises to anyone facing the difficulties a pituitary condition presents or, indeed, for anyone dealing with the stresses of life in general and to nurture and nourish ourselves, especially through more challenging periods. Besides making sure we are taking the correct dose of medication, there are activities that can help us remain positive, such as taking gentle walks, a relaxing break, enjoying a delicious meal, spending time with nature, family and friends, or doing anything that brings happiness and a sense of well-being. Living with a pituitary condition is, indeed, quite a journey for all patients. If you haven't already read The Pituitary Foundation's booklet, *Your Journey: Living and Managing a Pituitary Condition*,[13] then I know you will find it helpful and encouraging.

As the golden age of seventy looms large on the horizon, the thought of how I will cope as I get older has crossed my mind! In an article in Pituitary Life, Dr Sue Jackson[14] looks at the possible psychosocial aspects of getting older with a pituitary condition and refers to recent research which suggests there is a wide range of experiences of ageing in the normal population, both positive and negative and that it is probable that those with a pituitary condition will also either age well or experience difficulties. Problems that arise for older people may include poorer health, problems getting around, stigma and discrimination and loneliness. In the latter case it is helpful to remember that The Pituitary Foundation has a telephone buddy system that can help some of us feel less alone and misunderstood as we get older. I'm sure it isn't all bad and there are some things that can be done so that life continues to be interesting and worthwhile, such as attempting new learning experiences and staying active. However, as stated in the above article, there will be some pituitary patients who would find everyday living very tiring on its own without having to think about new learning experiences. Dr Jackson concludes that:

> ... there are large gaps in our knowledge about the
> psychosocial aspects of living with a pituitary condition
> ...

She goes on to mention a project being undertaken to improve our understanding of issues associated with young people who have a pituitary condition and suggests that:

> ... a similar project focussed on the needs of older
> adults would be very useful to help us develop a
> proper understanding of what it's like to age with a
> pituitary condition.

Such research would certainly be most welcome but, in the meantime, I would hope to remain as positive and as active as I can. With the continuing love and support of my husband, family and friends, I'm sure I will be able to carry on with optimism.

I'll always be grateful to the medical staff and therapists who have treated me, including those who continue to keep me going, both with my pituitary condition and my bone health. Although there will inevitably be times of sadness ahead and hurdles to leap over, I look forward to surprise events or those already planned, including our youngest daughter Rachel's wedding later this year. I'm already looking at hats for the second time!

I have often asked myself what I have learned from my

journey. Has it been a lesson in disguise to enable me to grow as a person, to be more aware of the needs of others, to love myself despite what has been going on with my body since November 1972? I've realised that it often takes an unexpected life-changing event, such as a diagnosis of a pituitary condition, to open the doors to acceptance of who we really are and learning that, despite the rough times life throws at us, we are all worthy, capable human beings. At the beginning of his book, *Cancer. My Personal Story*[15], my brother wrote that he felt lucky, not for the fact that he had cancer, but that whatever he suffered there would always be someone somewhere worse off. A brave statement and, whether a cliché of not, its truth has inspired me.

A few years ago I wrote this:

Today's gift is wrapped in blue with yellow ribbons.
As I untie them, the wrapper falls away revealing a box.
Inside are unknown treasures which will reveal themselves
with every passing second.
Mysteries to be unfolded and known.
I'll stack these unconsciously, on top of those of yesterday
And the day before that.
Going back into the past – taking me out into the future.

Appendix

The master gland

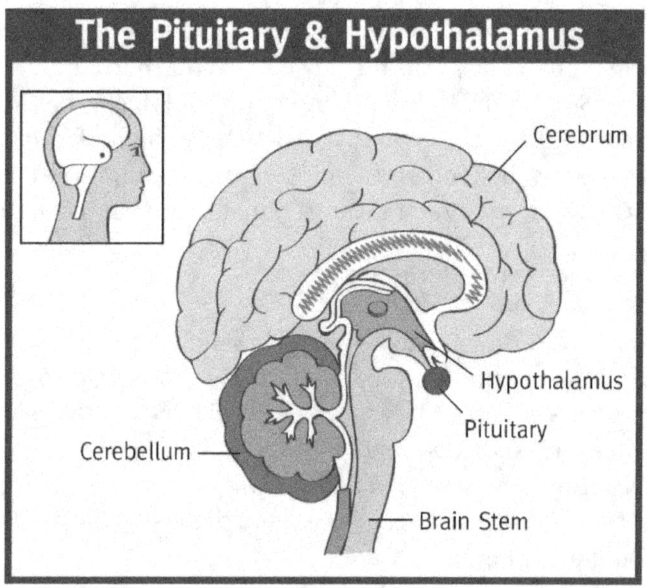

The pituitary gland is often referred to as the 'master gland', because it controls several of the other hormone glands, for example the adrenals and thyroid. It sits behind the bridge of the nose and below the base of the brain, close to the optic nerves. It never ceases to amaze me that this extraordinary gland, which produces hormones that control many functions of other endocrine glands, is usually the size of a large pea.

The endocrine system

The endocrine system consists of various glands situated in different parts of the body. Each gland produces different hormones (chemical messengers) which regulate the activity of other organs and tissues in the body. These hormones are released directly into the blood through the relevant gland.

The pituitary gland is made up of two sections, the anterior and posterior pituitary. In my case, the anterior pituitary became atrophied following the pituitary apoplexy which meant it could no longer produce hormones to stimulate the glands in my body to secrete their own hormones.

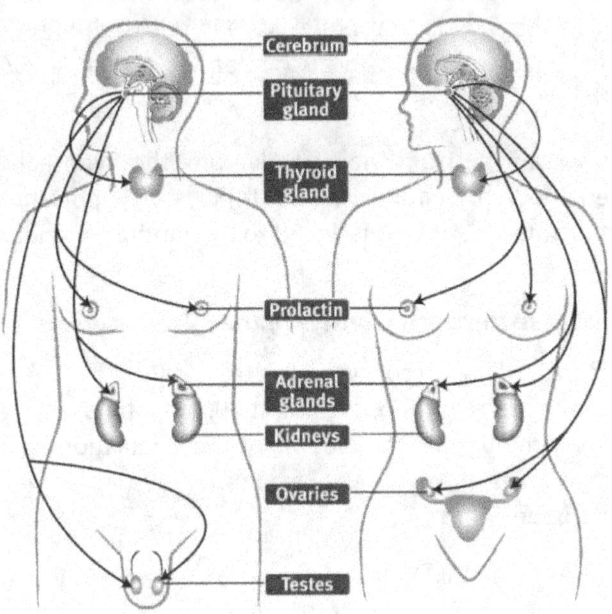

The endocrine system

One of the hormones normally produced by the anterior lobe is known as ACTH (adrenocorticotropic hormone) which targets the adrenals, stimulating them to produce cortisol. Others are: the thyroid-stimulating hormone (TSH), which stimulates the thyroid gland to secrete thyroxine; the luteinising hormone (LH), which controls the reproductive system; the follicle-stimulating hormone (FSH), which promotes the formation of ova or eggs in the ovary or sperm in men; prolactin (PRL), which causes milk to be produced after a baby is born; growth hormone (GH), which targets all cells in the body and stimulates growth and repair; and melanocyte-stimulating hormone (MSH) – the exact role of this hormone in humans is unknown.

My posterior pituitary was unaffected so that it continues to produce the anti-diuretic hormone (ADH), which tells my kidneys how much water to conserve, and oxytocin which is sometimes known as the 'cuddle hormone' as it is released when people snuggle up together. It is also released during labour and breastfeeding.

As you can see from the first diagram, the hypothalamus is situated above the pituitary gland. It plays an important role in the endocrine system and is linked to the pituitary gland.

Diseases and disorders of the pituitary gland

Pituitary disorders are considered rare. The Pituitary Foundation website reports that there are about 70,000 pituitary patients in the UK which equates to 0.0012% of the population, but some reports suggest as many as 1 in 5 may have an undiagnosed pituitary issue.

According to Wikipedia, there is only one study that has measured the prevalence (total number of cases alive in a population during a period of time) and incidence (annual number of new cases) of hypopituitarism. This study was conducted in Northern Spain and used hospital records in a well-defined population. The study showed that 45.5 people out of 100,000 had been diagnosed with hypopituitarism, with 4.2 new cases per year; 61% were due to tumours of the pituitary gland, 9% due to other types of lesions, and 19% due to other causes, in 11% no cause could be identified.

It would appear that the most common cause of hypopituitarism is a benign pituitary tumour, yet some pituitary tumours can exist for years without causing symptoms. The Pituitary Foundation website explains that 'the most common type of tumour is the "non" functioning' tumour which can cause headaches and visual problems or it can press on the pituitary gland, causing it to stop producing the required amount of one or more of the pituitary hormones.'

Common pituitary disorders besides hypopituitarism, include Acromegaly, Cushing's disease, diabetes insipidus, prolactinoma and adult growth hormone deficiency. Rarer disorders include Kallmann's syndrome, and Wolfram syndrome. I won't go into these or other pituitary disorders here but if you are interested in discovering more about them or anything summarised in this appendix, you can find what you need on The Pituitary Foundation website (www.pituitary.org.uk).

Apart from the reference to Wikipedia, the information and illustrations in this Appendix are courtesy of The Pituitary Foundation.

References

1. Rajasekaran, S., Vanderpump, M., Baldeweg, S. *et al.* (2011) UK guidelines for the management of pituitary apoplexy. *Clinical Endocrinology*, Volume 74, pages 9–20.This information is provided by the Society for Endocrinology's Clinical Committee, February 2013, and will be reviewed annually. If any changes occur a revised version will be made available. Revised February 2014. Society for Endocrinology, 22 Apex Court, Woodlands, Bradley Stoke, Bristol, BS32 4JT, UK.
2. The Pituitary Foundation website www.pituitary.org.uk.
3. *Pituitary Life*, Issue 15, July 2010.
4. Pat McBride, following a presentation at the recent Pituitary Conference, by Professor Richard Ross from the University of Sheffield. (2012) Tiredness and Fatigue in Hypopituitarism. *Pituitary Life*, Issue 20, pages 3-5
5. 'Hydrocortisone Advice for Pituitary Patient' leaflet published by The Pituitary Foundation.
6. Dr Aikaterini Theodoraki, SpR in Endocrinology and Diabetes Melitus and Dr Stephanie E Baldeweg, consultant physician in Diabetes & Endocrinology, Honorary Senior Lecturer UCLH, Department of Diabetes & Endocrinology, UCLH NHS Foundation Trust. (2013) How each hormone replacement medication may affect other hormone levels. *Pituitary Life*, Issue 25, pages 8–10.
7. Dr Trevor A Howlett, MD FRCP. Consultant Endocrinologist, Leicester Royal Infirmary. (2011) Make Hormones Count. *Pituitary Life*, Issue 19, pages 2-4
8. Angie Buxton-King. (2005) *The NHS Healer: how my son's life inspired a healing journey*. London: Virgin.
9. James L. Oschman, PhD. (2009) Nature's own research association, in Energy Medicine. The Scientific Basis. Dover, New Hampshire, USA. Churchill Livingstone, pages 177–8.
10. Susan E Brown, Ph.D, Director, Osteoporosis Education Project. *Better Bones, Better Body*. Beyond Estrogen and Calcium: comprehensive self-help programme for preventing, halting and overcoming osteoporosis. Second Edition. Los Angeles : Keats Pub., pages 374–6.
11. Ibid. Chapter 4, page 78 and Chapter 11, p 248
12. Ibid. Chapter 6, Page 146.
13. Your Journey: Living with and Managing a Pituitary Condition. The Pituitary Foundation. April 2013 version.
14. Dr Sue Jackson. (2015) The possible psychosocial aspects of getting older with a pituitary condition. *Pituitary Life*, Issue 30, pages 11–12, 21.
15. John Nelson. (2015) *Cancer. My Personal Story: Pulling the Positives out of the Negatives*. Available on Amazon (www.amazon.co.uk). All proceeds from the sale of this book go to Cancer Research.